D1488347

HOSPITAL PURCHASING AND INVENTORY MANAGEMENT

Edward D. Sanderson
St. Francis Hospital
Blue Island, Illinois

AN ASPEN PUBLICATION®
Aspen Systems Corporation
Rockville, Maryland
London
1982

Library of Congress Cataloging in Publication Data

Sanderson, Edward D.
Hospital purchasing and inventory management.

Includes index.
1. Hospitals— Materials management.
2. Hospitals— Purchasing.
I. Title.
[DNLM: 1. Purchasing, Hospital. 2. Materials
management, Hospital. WX 157 S216h]
RA971.33.S36   362.1'1'0687   81-12733
ISBN: 0-89443-389-X   AACR2

Copyright © 1982 Aspen Systems Corporation

Library of Congress Catalog Card Number: 81-12733
ISBN: 0-89443-389-X

Printed in the United States of America

2 3 4 5

To my wife, *Donna*

Table of Contents

Preface

In 1979, the General Accounting Office released the results of a study of hospital purchasing practices, entitled "Study of Purchasing and Materials Management Functions in Private Hospitals." This study was critical of many of our practices, but it was constructive criticism. The study was beneficial inasmuch as it commended hospitals that utilized good procedures and pointed out flaws in procedures that required correction.

Of the 21 test hospitals, and particularly the four intensively audited hospitals, each received both favorable and unfavorable comments regarding its practices. The examples cited throughout the study are real. I know because I was the director of materials management at one of the four intensively audited hospitals.

When I read the final report, I concurred with the conclusion that the results applied to hospitals nationwide. The inevitable question was "Why?" I did not find immediate answers. It was not until I was approached about writing this book that I began to seek the answers in earnest. Everywhere I turned, and from everyone with whom I spoke, the reply was the same: Growth! The acceptance of the materiel management concept had grown so fast that it was siphoning qualified purchasing practitioners to meet the demand.

Because of the growth of the materiel management concept, hospitals began to promote untrained people from within—people with little or no formal training in basic procedures. Secretaries became buyers overnight, and there simply was no time to teach them properly. In an effort to supplement the available supply, hospitals began hiring people from industry. These people were not familiar with hospital routine. And the problem compounded itself because there were few, if any, nontheoretical references available to provide answers to their questions—answers that many "experienced" practitioners had little time to give. It is for these "forgotten" people that this book is intended.

This text should be useful to experienced as well as inexperienced practitioners, educators, and students, and should fill the void for a practical, nontheoretical handbook on hospital purchasing practices and techniques. And if just one person involved in hospital purchasing finds some beneficial use for the material contained in this book, it will have been worth the effort.

Edward D. Sanderson, C.H.P.M.
December 1981

Acknowledgments

I would like to express my appreciation and gratitude to the administrations and staffs of Delnor Hospital, St. Charles, Illinois, and St. Francis Hospital, Blue Island, Illinois. Without their support, encouragement, and cooperation, this work would not have been possible.

To John A. Taft, Jr., Bryant R. Hanson, and Edward L. Rosen, a special thanks for believing and trusting in my abilities and for allowing me to implement many of these procedures in their respective hospitals.

I also owe a special debt of gratitude to a colleague and good friend, William Klee. His concern, encouragement, and review of this material greatly improved my ability to write this book.

And a special thanks to my wife, Donna, whose typing, proofing, and faith in my ability were invaluable.

Chapter 1
Designing a Purchasing System

Basic to any purchasing operation is the communication by an individual or department of the need for specific goods and services and the transmission of information concerning those needs to the proper vendor. To accomplish the process successfully, the purchasing practitioner should utilize a systematic approach to information processing.

A sound purchasing system is one that will provide for (1) a uniform purchase order, (2) proper documentation of all purchases, and (3) a uniform accounts payable procedure to ensure proper payment. (See Exhibit 1-1 for an example of purchase order control procedures.) Regardless of whether the hospital has a centralized or decentralized purchasing system (with pharmacy and dietary doing their own purchasing in the latter), there should be uniformity of documentation and processing.

A basic purchasing system consists of four documents: a purchase requisition, a purchase order, a change order, and a return material/credit memorandum. Serving as a foundation, these four documents will provide for the successful flow of information and documentation necessary to carry out the purchasing function.

The purchasing forms system detailed in this chapter is provided as a guide to the reader. Each of the exampled forms has been designed to complement each of the others, and yet is distinctive enough to provide recognition of its function within the system.

PURCHASE REQUISITION

Despite the fact that the practitioner has the law of agency, most hospitals employ some type of budgeting procedure whereby department heads are responsible for supplies and equipment charged to their departmental budgets. Where such a budget system is employed, the purchasing practitioner must have some

Exhibit 1-1 Purchase Order Control Procedure

```
                                                        Procedure
                                                        MMPD-006
                                                        2/7/80

                        ST. FRANCIS HOSPITAL
                        BLUE ISLAND, ILLINOIS


                    MATERIEL MANAGEMENT DEPARTMENT
                         PURCHASING DIVISION
                        PURCHASE ORDER CONTROL


                              POLICY

        Purchasing shall issue a purchase order for all procurements
        and commitments.



                             PURPOSE

        To provide a method of documentation for all purchase orders.



                            PROCEDURE

        I. A purchase order log book will be maintained to record
        all purchase order numbers issued.

                A. This log will be maintained in consecutive number
                   sequence inorder to account for all purchase orders.

                B. The purchase order log (attachment A) will be completed
                   as follows:

                   1. P.O.# - enter purchase order number

                   2. Company - enter company name

                   3. Department - enter name of department for whom
                                   merchandise ordered. For p.o.'s
                                   with multiple departments enter
                                   the word various.


                   4. Date - enter order date

                   5. Total Amount P.O. - enter the total dollar amount
                                          for all items on the p.o.

                   6. Total Line Items - enter total line items listed
                                         on the purchase order

                   7. Ordered By - enter initials of individual placing
                                   the order.
```

Exhibit 1-1 continued

II. At the end of the month, a summary of all purchase orders written will be submitted to the Director, Materiel Management. This report will include:

    A. Total Purchase Orders Written
    B. Total Line Items
    C. Total Dollar Value - excluding Capital Equipment

III. The department secretary is responsible to maintain the purchase order log and submit the monthly report.

_____
Purchasing Manager

_____
Director, Materiel Management

type of supporting documentation to authorize purchases charged to any given department's budget. Purchasing should never be allowed to process purchase orders, except for supplies for the department itself, without such authorization. The two most popular methods for departments to initiate an order are the traveling requisition and the direct purchase requisition.

In general, the traveling requisition is used for items with a high recurrence of reorder. Exhibit 1-2 is a sample of this form. Central stores, central service, laboratory, maintenance, radiology, and surgery are typical examples of departments that could make good use of the traveling requisition.

The traveling requisition is normally exchanged between the ordering department and purchasing (thus its name). Central stores' use of the traveling requisition will naturally correspond to the items maintained in the inventory. Each traveling requisition is marked with the corresponding catalog or item stock number. (This is discussed further in Chapter 10.)

Exhibit 1-2 Traveling Requisition

ITEM DESCRIPTION

STOCK NO.

HOW PACKAGED: UNIT OF ISSUE:

MFG'S STOCK NUMBER

CODE	VENDORS	ADDRESS	CITY	STATE	ZIP	PHONE	DELIVER TO	ACCT. NO.	VENDOR NO.
1									
2									
3									
4									

PRICE SCHEDULE

VENDOR	QTY.	PRICE	UNITS	DATE	TERMS	F. O. B.	PRICE CHGE.	DATE
1								
2								
3								
4								

ANNUAL USAGE   **REMARKS**

YEAR: UNITS: LAST BID DATE

E.O.Q.   BID NUMBER

REORDER PT.   STD. COST:

PURCHASE RECORD

DATE	QTY.	UNIT	REQUESTED BY	DATE ORDERED	VENDOR P. O. NO.	QTY./UNIT	PRICE	TOTAL COST	ORD'D BY	REMARKS

The traveling requisition offers a number of advantages:

1. a reduction in paperwork and associated purchasing costs
2. uniform commodity information (pricing, standard ordering units, vendor information, etc.)
3. centralized and continuous purchase history
4. automatic listing of authorized substitutes

The last point is particularly important in that it provides a basis for future negotiation and inventory control decisions.

The traveling requisition also has disadvantages:

1. Departments with a large number of traveling requisitions may require significant clerical effort to maintain the necessary files.
2. Some departments may encounter the need for additional reorder while the traveling requisition is in transit between departments.

Although this second problem seldom arises, it still must be recognized. Depending upon the frequency of occurrence, a second card might be employed, but this is not recommended as standard practice. Should the problem surface on a regular basis for a particular item, a thorough review should be undertaken to explore such potential remedies as recalculation of the reorder point and stocking in central stores.

When a traveling requisition is utilized for ordering purposes, the information it contains must be converted to a purchase order. This information conversion must be understood by all personnel who come into contact with it in the course of their duties.

The upper portion of the card contains all of the relevant information to describe the item and the potential vendor from whom it may be purchased. This particular portion of the requisition is for the use of the practitioner to maintain current information.

The lower portion ("Purchase Record") contains information provided by the requisitioner and completed by the practitioner. The left side of the card is completed by the requisitioner and simply requires the date the order is initiated, the quantity and unit desired, and a signature in the column headed "Requested by." The remainder of the lower section is used by the practitioner to record the date of the order, vendor, purchase order number, quantity and unit ordered, price per unit, total cost, and the initials of the person placing the order.

When the requisition is received by the typist, the information on the last completed line under the heading "Purchase Record" is used to prepare the purchase order. Information is extracted from the requisition to correspond with the requirements of the purchase order.

Direct Purchase Requisition

The second method of initiating an order is the direct purchase requisition. This form is used by all departments for one-time or nonrecurring purchases and for capital equipment. Exhibit 1-3 is a typical example of the direct purchase requisition. As you will note, the direct purchase requisition includes adequate space for the requisitioner to provide all the information necessary to complete a purchase. The right-hand side of the direct purchase requisition is used for normal purchasing information that is relevant to preparing the purchase order. Space has been provided for the purchase order number, date ordered, name of person placing the order, terms of payment, FOB, delivery, and how the order was transmitted. Also included is space for information regarding capital equipment purchases. As with any form, the desired information will vary with each hospital's requirements. Finally, space is provided for a suggested vendor, as well as for department head and/or administrative approval.

Information on the direct purchase requisition is converted to a purchase order almost exactly as it is detailed on the requisition. The practitioner is responsible for noting any corrections necessary to permit a clear statement of the transaction so that the information appearing on the purchase order will be clearly understood by all who must read it.

The direct purchase requisition recommended (Exhibit 1-3) is a four-part form. Each part performs a specific, singular function in the communication process. The top copy (part 1, identified as "purchasing") is attached to purchasing's copy of the purchase order and serves as the necessary documentation for authorization of the purchase.

The second copy (identified as "accounting") is attached to accounting's copy of the purchase order and acts as a source document to allocate funds and charge the purchase to the originating department's budget.

The third copy (identified as "purchasing") is used to establish a record of the purchase by the particular department. This file is maintained by the purchasing department to provide a basis for research to (1) determine if a recurring purchase situation exists, (2) find a record of an item purchased for the particular department without knowing the vendor from whom it was purchased, and (3) provide an information base for future commodity negotiations.

The fourth copy (identified as "department") provides the originating department with a copy of the request to be used for followup or some other reference. Often, the fact that the originator retains a copy of the requisition can lead to the elimination of duplicate orders.

Exhibit 1-3 Direct Purchase Requisition

ST. FRANCIS HOSPITAL
BLUE ISLAND, ILLINOIS

DIRECT PURCHASE REQUISITION

THIS IS NOT A
PURCHASE ORDER

DEPARTMENT

DATE OF REQUEST

DELIVERY DATE REQUIRED

REQUEST INITIATED BY

ACCOUNT NUMBER

USE SEPARATE REQUISITIONS FOR EACH VENDOR.
ORDERS WILL BE PROCESSED WHEN ALL REQUIRED INFORMATION IS COMPLETED.

QUANTITY	UNIT	VENDOR ITEM NUMBER	DESCRIPTION OF ITEMS	UNIT PRICE	PURCHASING USE ONLY

SUGGESTED

VENDOR
AND
ADDRESS

DEPARTMENT HEAD
APPROVAL

ADMINISTRATIVE
APPROVAL

FOR PURCHASING'S USE ONLY

VENDOR

PURCHASE ORDER NO

DATE

ORDERED BY

TERMS

F O B

DELIVERY

CALL   SALESMAN
MAIL   CONFIRMED

DATE

CONTACT

CAPITAL BUDGET
IF THIS IS A CAPITAL EXPENDITURE IS
IT INCLUDED IN THE APPROVED BUDGET?

YES   NO

REVIEWED BY:

PLANT ENGR _____ DATE _____

CLIN ENGR

OTHER _____ DATE _____

PURCHASE ORDER

The purchase order is the vehicle with which the buyer formalizes the purchase with the vendor. In almost every instance, the purchase order is a legal document and must contain all elements required for a contract. The purchase order may be simple or complex. Regardless of its design, it must contain all of the elements necessary to describe the purchase or transaction (Exhibit 1-4). The items necessary for inclusion are as follows:

Masthead. The masthead includes the hospital name, address, Zip code, and telephone number. If the ship-to address or billing address is different from the hospital's mailing address, that fact should be noted in this area.

Purchase Order Number. For control purposes all purchase orders should be prenumbered. The purchase order number will be used for receiving and invoicing purposes.

Seller's Name. This area should include the full name and address of the vendor. Normally, the original copy of the purchase order is sent or given to the vendor for record-keeping purposes.

Date of Order. There are two schools of thought concerning this area. Some practitioners believe that the date the verbal order is given should appear here regardless of when the order is typed. Others hold that the date the order is typed should be indicated.

If a verbal order is placed with a vendor with a confirming purchase order to follow, the date of the order must be the same as the date of the verbal commitment. Under contract law, in order for the prior oral agreement to be a binding contract, the followup written agreement (your purchase order) must satisfy the requirement of definiteness. If it does not, it may mean that there was no oral agreement, and thus no contract. This point is clarified further in Chapter 4.

Date Required. This area is used for the delivery date.

Terms. Some vendors offer discounts for prompt payment; others do not. In either case, the payment terms of the agreement should be entered. Normally, abbreviations such as 2 percent—10; net 30 will suffice.

Ship Via. Any special shipping instructions should be noted in this area; for example, your truck, United Parcel Service, first class mail, parcel post.

FOB. This abbreviation for "free on board" refers to the point of delivery of the merchandise by the vendor. FOB also determines the point at which title to the merchandise passes from the vendor to the hospital. Usually, damages sustained prior to the FOB point are the responsibility of the vendor whereas damages sustained after that point are the responsibility of the hospital. Each is responsible for filing claims for damage according to the FOB point.

Exhibit 1-4 Purchase Order

☾f ST. FRANCIS HOSPITAL

12935 South Gregory Street   Blue Island, Illinois 60406

312-597-2000

PURCHASE ORDER NO.	PO-

THE ABOVE NUMBER MUST APPEAR ON ALL CARTONS, INVOICES, SHIPPING DOCUMENTS AND CORRESPONDENCE RELATIVE TO THIS ORDER.

PLEASE ENTER OUR ORDER FOR THE FOLLOWING ITEMS: SUBJECT TO ALL CONDITIONS ON THE FACE AND BACK OF THIS ORDER.

TERMS AND CONDITIONS

It is requested that packing slip be securely attached to exterior of shipping carton.

This Order may not be modified or changed, orally or in any other manner, except in writing signed by the authorized representative of the Purchasing Department.

All merchandise must be delivered to Receiving between 8:00 A.M. - 4:00 P.M.

Transportation charges shall be prepaid to point of delivery specified, and add to invoice. Any prepaid charges must be supported at time of invoice by freight or express receipts including Hospital purchase order number.

Acceptance of all goods and materials furnished under this Order are subject to buyers inspection at point of use. Payment for materials delivered prior to inspection shall not constitute acceptance thereof.

The buyers reserve the right to return any or all items not deemed acceptable for any reason by mutual agreement and in compliance with seller policy regarding returns.

The delivery date of items involved with construction must be confirmed with the Purchasing Office. 5 working days before delivery. Any deliveries on this purchase order must be confirmed 5 working days before delivery if the items require a mechanical or construction connection to the building.

It shall be the responsibility of the seller to arrange for returning items shipped in error or duplication at no cost to the buyer in a period of time not exceeding normal delivery shall be rendered.

The seller must advise the buyer by return mail of extended delivery times or back order situations of items in this order.

Non-compliance with the instructions and conditions of this Order will be cause for refusal of shipment.

St. Francis Hospital is a non-profit institution exempt from the Retailers' Occupation Tax and the Service Occupation Tax and the Service Use Tax.

We will not be responsible for goods or services delivered or rendered except on a properly authorized Purchase Order.

This Purchase Order is subject to all terms and conditions as shown on the face and back.

DATE OF ORDER	DATE REQUIRED	TERMS	SHIP VIA	F. O. B.	DEPARTMENT

ITEM NO.	QUANTITY	UNIT	DESCRIPTION	CODING DEPT.	CODING ACCT.	PRICE PER UNIT	AMOUNT
						TOTAL	

BY _____

AUTHORIZED SIGNATURE

The FOB point is often a source of confusion. Therefore, a simple explanation is offered.

- FOB Hospital. Under normal conditions, this is usually the most advantageous for the hospital. The vendor absorbs all transportation costs and must file all claims for damages.

- FOB Shipping Point. Here, the vendor ships by common carrier and title passes to the hospital at the time of shipping. The hospital pays the freight charges and files all claims for damages.

- FOB Shipping Point, Freight Prepaid. Title passes to the hospital when the merchandise is picked up by the carrier, but the vendor prepays the freight charges and adds the cost to the invoice. The hospital files all damage claims.

- FOB Shipping Point, Freight Allowed. Title passes to the hospital when the merchandise is picked up by the carrier, but the vendor reimburses the hospital for shipping costs.

Clarification of the FOB point is important since responsibility for damages must be clear. Also, transportation costs can become a significant factor in the total cost of the item(s) ordered. For this reason, every effort should be made to utilize FOB Hospital. When this cannot be done, freight charges should be specified as to basic rate costs and total freight costs. The total freight costs should be reflected as a separate item on the purchase order and included in the total cost.

Department. This is used to identify the ordering department(s).

Quantity/Unit. This area provides for clear delineation of the exact quantity and unit of measure of the item(s) ordered. Care must be taken to provide clear and concise information to be used by both the vendor and accounting in completing the transaction.

Description. Again, clear and concise information is necessary. Use of product code number, size, proper nouns, and quantity per unit of measure are necessary to help reduce the possibility for error in the various stages of the transaction that are to follow. The following is an example of such descriptive information.

Gloves, surgeon's, latex, sterile, white, size 6, Arbrook #5860, 50 pairs/box, 4 boxes/case

Practitioners should establish this type of standard for providing product information. All parties to the transaction (vendor, accounting, receiving, etc.) should be informed and have a clear understanding of the standard provided.

Price per Unit and Amount. A standard practice should be established to price and extend (amount) all purchase orders prior to forwarding to the vendor. If you are working from a quotation or a group contract, you are accepting an offer made by the vendor. Your acceptance of the offer should include the agreed upon price.

If you are purchasing an item without a written quotation or contract (i.e., working from a price list), you are making the offer to buy from the vendor. Your offer must include the price you are willing to pay for the merchandise. Failure to include a price gives the vendor your implied consent to pay whatever price the vendor wishes to charge.

The purchase price and total extension will also aid the vendor in processing an invoice, as well as provide your accounting department with an accurate method to verify the vendor's invoice. The unit price and extended amount act as a complete summary of the purchasing transaction.

Care must be taken to ensure that the price per unit is in agreement with the unit of measure. A common mistake made by purchasing practitioners is to order an item by the case and use the per-item price, which often results in extension errors. This type of mistake can be illustrated using an order for one case of surgeon's gloves, four boxes per case, at $79.24 per case.

Incorrect:

Qty	Unit	Description	Unit Cost	Total Cost
1	cs	Gloves, surgeon's, size 6 Arbrook # 5860, 4 bx/cs	$19.81	$19.81

Correct:

Qty	Unit	Description	Unit Cost	Total Cost
1	cs	Gloves, surgeon's, size 6 Arbrook # 5860, 4 bx/cs	$79.24	$79.24

With this illustration, the incorrect example uses the price per box and results in a $59.43 error. Care and consistency are a matter of fact, not of choice.

Terms and Conditions. It has been said that the terms and conditions or "boilerplate" of the hospital purchase order are notorious—notoriously bad, that is. Corporations go to great lengths to ensure that the terms and conditions of their purchase orders and quotation forms afford protection for the company. To accomplish this, companies hire contract attorneys to provide the proper wherefores and therefores. In many hospitals, the purchasing practitioner attains, or is thrust into, this position.

Terms and conditions are not something to fear or to ignore. As the agent for the hospital, the purchasing practitioner is responsible for safeguarding the interests of the hospital. To that end, the practitioner should be familiar with the Uniform Commercial Code as it applies to contracts and sales of merchandise and services. (See Exhibit 1-5 for an example of a terms and conditions document.)

Exhibit 1-5 Terms and Conditions

BUYER'S TERMS AND CONDITIONS
OF PURCHASE AS AMENDED 1/80

1. ACCEPTANCE: This order is for the purchase and sale of the goods (herein referred to as "the Articles") and/or services described on the attached purchase order and is the Hospital's offer to Seller. Acknowledgement hereof by Seller to Buyer shall consitute Seller's acceptance of such order, including all of the terms and conditions herein set out. In the absence of such acknowledgement, commencement of delivery of the Articles and/or services and acceptance of such deliveries by Buyer shall consitute a firm contract on the terms and conditions hereof. This order is subject to the following terms and conditions and no others unless there is a signed overriding agreement between the parties prepared by Hospital.

2. PACKING: The Articles shall be packed and shipped by Seller in accordance with Hospital's instructions and good commercial practice and so as to insure that no damage shall result from weather or transportation.

3. WARRANTY-PRODUCT: Seller warrants that all the Articles will be free from defects in material and workmanship, will conform to specifications, drawings and other descriptions and to accepted samples and, if ordered for a stated purpose, will be fit for such purpose. Seller also warrants that to the extent the Articles are not manufactured pursuant to detailed designs furnished by Hospital they will be free from defects in design, and agrees to make such changes, adjustments, or replacements as necessary to meet the guarantee, at no cost to the Hospital. Such warranties, including warranties prescribed by law, shall run to Hospital, its successors, assigns and heirs, and to users of the Articles, for a period of one year after delivery of such longer period as may be prescribed by law or additional agreement.

4. WARRANTY-PRICE: Seller warrants that prices that are charged Hospital, as indicated on the front side hereof, are no higher than prices charged on orders placed by others for similar conditions subsequent to the last general announced price change. In the event Seller breaches this warranty, the prices of the Articles shall be reduced accordingly retroactive to date of such breach.

5. TERMINATION:

   a. Hospital may cancel this order, in whole or in part, without liability to Hospital, if deliveries are not made at the time and the quantities or conditions hereof.

   b. Hospital may terminate this order in whole or part at any time for its convenience by notice to Seller in writing. On receipt by Seller of such notice, Seller shall, and to the extent specified therein, stop work hereunder and the placements of subcontracts, terminate work under subcontracts outstanding hereunder, and take

Exhibit 1-5 continued

any necessary action to protect property in Seller's possession in which Hospital has or may acquire an interest. Any termination claim must be submitted to Hospital within sixty (60) days after effective date of termination.

  c. Any cancellation or termination by Hospital, whether for default or otherwise, shall be without prejudice to any claims for damages or other rights of Hospital against Seller.

  d. Hospital may cancel this order, in whole or in part, without liability to Hospital, if deliveries are not made at the time and in the quantities specified or in the event of a breach or failure of any of the other terms or conditions hereof.

6. CHANGES: Hospital at any time may make changes in the quantities ordered or in the specifications of drawings relating to the Articles or may exchange or amend any other term or condition of this order, in which event an equitable adjustment will be made to any price, time of performance and/or other provisions of this order required to be changed thereby. Any claim for such an adjustment must be made within fifteen (15) days from date of receipt by Seller of such change.

7. COMPLIANCE WITH LAWS: In filling this order, Seller shall comply with all applicable federal, state and local laws and goverment regulations and orders. Seller specifically warrants and guarantees to Hospital:

  a. that the Articles are in compliance with Sections 5 and 12 of the Federal Trade Commission Act, and are properly labeled as to content as required by applicable Federal Trade Commission Trade Practice Rules;

  b. that all Articles furnished hereunder will be produced and sold in compliance with all applicable requirements of the Fair Labor Standards Act, as amended, including Sections 6, 7, and 12, and the regulations and orders issued under Section 14, thereof, and that it will certify such compliance on each invoice submitted in connection with this order;

  c. that the Articles are in compliance with the Consumer Product Safety Act of 1972;

  d. that the Articles are not manufactured or sold in violation of the Occupational Safety and Health Act of 1970;

  e. that the Articles are not manufactured or sold in violation of the Medical Device Amendments of 1976.

Exhibit 1-5 continued

8. INDEMNITY AND INSURANCE:

    a. Seller shall defend, indemnify and hold harmless Hospital, its employees and users of the Articles, from and against any claim, loss, damage or expense arising out of the purchase and/or use of the Articles purchased hereunder and/or arising out of Seller's (or its subcontractos's) work or performance hereunder and shall procure and maintain liability insurance, with contractural liability coverage, with minimum limits of $250,000/ $500,000/$100,000or such higher limits as Hospital shall reasonably request. Seller shall, on or before delivery of the Articles purchased hereunder, furnish to Hospital a Certificate of Insurance evidencing the foregoing coverages and limits.

    b. Seller shall defend, indemnify and hold harmless Hospital from and against the assessment by any third party of any liquidated damages or proven actual damages arising out of the failure of Seller to timely deliver the Articles purchased hereunder.

    c. Seller shall defend, indemnify and hold harmless Hospital, its employees and users of the Articles from and against any claim loss (Including the cost of any Articles lost by libel, condemnation or voluntary recall), damage arising out of any claim or finding by the United States of America or any state or local government or any agency or instrumentality thereof that the Articles are not herein guaranteed and warranted.

9. ASSIGNMENT: Seller shall not assign this order or any interest herein, including any performance or any amount which may be due or may become due hereunder, without Hospital's prior written consent.

10. SUBCONTRACTING: If any Articles are to be made to Hospital's design, and/or services described on the front hereof, all subcontracting by Seller with respect thereto shall be subject to Hospital's written approval which shall not be indescriminately withheld.

11. ADVERTISING: Seller shall not advertise or publish the fact that Hospital has placed this order without Hospital's prior written consent except as may be necessary to comply with a proper request for information from an authorized representative of any government unit or agency.

12. CONTROLLING LAW: This order and the performance of the parties hereunder shall be controlled and governed by the law of the state shown in Hospital's address on the front side hereof.

13. NOTICE OF LABOR DISPUTES: Whenever an actual or potential labor dispute is delaying or threatens to delay the timely performance of this order, Seller shall immediately give

Exhibit 1-5 continued

```
    notice thereof, including all relevant information with
    respect thereto, to Hospital. Seller shall insert the
    substance of this paragraph in any subcontract hereunder
    so that each subcontract shall provide that in the event its
    timely performance is delayed or threatened by delay by any
    actual or potential labor dispute, the subcontractor shall
    immediately notify Seller of all relevant information with
    respect to such dispute.

14. RISK OF LOSS:  Risk of loss or damage to the Articles shall
    be on Seller until said Articles have been delivered to
    and accepted by Hospital notwithstanding any other terms
    contained herein.  All Articles will be received by Hospital
    subject to its right of inspection and rejection.  Hospital
    shall be allowed a reasonable period of time to inspect
    the Articles and to notify Seller of any nonconformance with
    the terms and conditions of this order.  Hospital may reject
    any Articles which do not conform to the terms and conditions
    of this order.  Articles so rejected may be returned to Seller,
    or held by Hospital, at Seller's risk and expense.

15. GENERAL:  All warranties shall be construed as conditions as
    well as warranties.  No waiver of a breach or of any provisions
    of this order shall constitute a waiver of any other breach
    or provision.  No modification, change in, or departure from,
    or waiver of the provisions of this order shall be valid
    or binding unless approved by Hospital in writing.  This order
    shall constitute the entire agreement between the parties.
```

The terms and conditions contained on the hospital's purchase order should cover the following topics:

- acceptance
- packing
- warranty—product
- warranty—price
- termination
- changes
- compliance with laws

- indemnity and insurance
- assignment
- subcontracting
- advertising
- controlling law
- notice of labor disputes
- risk of loss

Whatever boilerplate is developed, the hospital attorney should approve it prior to its inclusion on the purchase order.

Purchase Order Distribution. The number of copies of the purchase order required will vary with each hospital. The purchasing practitioner should review this item at least annually.

The most common parts of the purchase order are as follows:

1. Vendor copy. This copy is self-explanatory and is often the most abused. Many purchasing practitioners have developed a habit of not sending confirming orders to the vendors. The reason given most often is to avoid duplicate shipments, and this is often a truism. However, under the Uniform Commercial Code, contracts with a value of $500 or more must be transmitted in writing.[1] Because of the terms and conditions on the purchase order, it is recommended that the vendor copy of the purchase order be sent to the vendor. The use of a large rubber stamp with the words "Confirming Order, Do Not Duplicate" is also recommended. Remember, mistakes and misunderstandings can happen over the telephone. If duplicate shipments do become a problem, sit down with your vendor representative and explain the necessity for the procedure. Have the representative ask the company's order department or customer service department to be on the alert for the confirmation copy.

2. Vendor acknowledgment. Many hospitals include an acknowledgment copy of the purchase order. This copy provides the purchasing department with an acceptance of the offer as made. Exceptions to the order by the vendor are usually made via this copy. The acknowledgment copy also provides assurance to the buyer that the order has been received and is being processed.

3. Purchasing. Some hospitals prefer to have two copies of the purchase order. One copy is maintained in the open order file until completed. The second copy is usually maintained in a numerical file to permit proper accounting of all purchase orders used. If a second copy of the purchase order is not desirable, a purchase order log may be substituted. Exhibit 1-6 is an example of a typical purchase order log. As noted, there is adequate space for the purchase order number, vendor name, department(s) the item(s) were ordered for, date the order was placed, total amount of the purchase order, total line items, who placed the order, and any applicable remarks.

4. Accounting. Accounting should receive a copy of the purchase order to allow proper invoice verification, payment, and voucher authorization.

5. Department. It is recommended that a copy of the purchase order be sent to the department(s) whose supplies or equipment have been ordered. This copy acts as an acknowledgment to the requesting department that its requisition has been received and an order placed. This copy also provides the requesting department with a reference for future followup action if that becomes necessary.

Exhibit 1-6 Purchase Order Log

P.O. #	COMPANY	DEPARTMENT	DATE	AMOUNT P.O	TOTAL LINES	ORDEREDBY	REMARKS

6. Receiving. Receiving usually has two copies of the purchase order—one for purchasing, and the other for accounts payable. Both copies are used to indicate receipts of the merchandise ordered and to show completion of the transaction by the vendor. Accounting will utilize its copy to verify the quantities received against the quantities shown on the vendor's invoice.

PURCHASE ORDER CHANGE NOTICE

This form is used to record any change(s) made to the original purchase order regardless of whether the change was initiated by the hospital or by the vendor. The purchasing practitioner should make it a strict policy that any and all changes to a purchase order be made in writing on a purchase order change notice (Exhibit 1-7). Even if a change was made orally, this form will acknowledge it, providing proper documentation and noting when the change was made and who authorized it.

The purchase order change notice should be completed in quadruplicate, with copies for the vendor, accounts payable, purchasing, and receiving. A fifth copy for the requesting department is optional. Typical changes on this form include price, unit of measure, FOB, quantity, and delivery date. (See Exhibit 1-8 for an example of purchase order change notice procedure.)

The mechanics of the change order system are uncomplicated and easily understood. The vendor copy is used either to notify the vendor of a hospital-initiated change or to confirm the hospital's recognition of a change requested by the vendor.

Accounting utilizes its copy of the form to update the original purchase order for payment processing purposes.

Receiving's copy is used to update the original purchase order properly to accomplish the necessary receiving procedures of check-in and distribution.

Purchasing employs its copy to update the original purchase order for complete documentation of the transaction.

Internal hospital departments should use identical procedures for updating or correcting the original purchase order. Changes made via the change order should be noted on the department's copy of the original purchase order. The change order form itself should be attached to the original copy of the purchase order and retained for documentation and reference purposes.

RETURN MATERIAL/CREDIT MEMORANDUM

With the large number of purchase orders processed by the hospital and the vendor, mistakes are bound to occur. Shipment of incorrect merchandise, discovery of hidden damage, and overshipments and invoice corrections are but a few of the problems that create a need for this type of form. As with the purchase order,

Exhibit 1-7 Purchase Order Change Notice

NO. _____

ST. FRANCIS HOSPITAL
12935 South Gregory Street
Blue Island, Illinois 60406

PURCHASE ORDER CHANGE NOTICE

DATE OF CHANGE	PURCHASE ORDER NUMBER	DATED	ADDRESS COMMUNICATIONS TO
			PURCHASING

Changes:	Item #	FROM	TO
Price ☐			
F.O.B. ☐			
Quantity ☐			
Specs. ☐			
Delivery ☐			
Cancel ☐			
Sub/Acct. Cost Center ☐			
☐			
☐		OLD TOTAL _____	NEW TOTAL _____

REMARKS:

CONFIRMING ☐ YES ☐ NO

TO:

_____
Purchasing

All terms and conditions of the Original Purchase
Order remain in effect, except as charged herein.

Exhibit 1-8 Purchase Order Change Notice Procedure

```
                                              PROCEDURE
                                              MMPD-007
                                              2/7/80

                    ST. FRANCIS HOSPITAL
                    BLUE ISLAND, ILLINOIS


                 MATERIEL MANAGEMENT DEPARTMENT
                       PURCHASING DIVISION
                 PURCHASE ORDER CHANGE NOTICE

                            POLICY
        Purchasing shall issue a purchase order for all procurements
        and commitments.

                           PURPOSE
        To provide a method of documentation for changes to the
        original purchase order.

                          PROCEDURE

        I.  A Purchase Order Change Notice will be used to record
            all changes to a previously written purchase order.

        II. The Purchase Order Change Notice will be completed
            as follows:

            1.  NO. (upper right hand corner)- enter the purchase
                order number and the change.  (example - 53122-1)

            2.  DATE OF CHANGE - enter date change is effective

            3.  PURCHASE ORDER NUMBER - enter original purchase
                order number

            4.  DATED - enter date of original purchase order

            5.  ADDRESS COMMUNICATION TO - enter name of person
                effecting change

            6.  CHANGES - place an "X" in the box which appropriately
                identifies the change being made.  For changes not
                identified, use any of two blank spaces at bottom
                of column.

            7.  ITEM # - enter item number from original purchase
                order

            8.  FROM - This area is to be used to identify
                original information on the purchase order.  For
                those changes which effect the unit on total cost,
                enter original purchase order total in the space
                marked "OLD TOTAL".

            9.  TO - This area is to be used to identify the new
                information.  For those changes which effect the
                unit on total cost, enter the new purchase order
                total in a space marked "NEW TOTAL".
```

Exhibit 1-8 continued

```
        10.  REMARKS - enter any additional information relating
             to the reason for the change

        11.  TO (inside boxed area, lower left) - enter vendor
             name and address

        12.  CONFIRMING - check appropriate box

        13.  _____ - enter signature of person
                  PURCHASING          authorizing the change

   III.  The Purchase Order Change Notice shall be distributed
         as follows:

         PART 1 - white - To Vendor
         PART 2 - canary - To Accounting
         PART 3 - pink - attach to Purchasing's copy of original
                         purchase order
         PART 4 - goldenrod - To Receiving


    _____
    PURCHASING MANAGER


    _____
    DIRECTOR, MATERIEL MANAGEMENT
```

clear and concise information is a necessity. After all, the hospital wants to receive full credit for the merchandise returned. Exhibit 1-9 is a sample of this form. This should also be a four-part form, with copies for the vendor, accounts payable, purchasing, and receiving. A fifth copy can be advantageous as it can be used as a packing slip for the returned merchandise.

The return material/credit memorandum provides for a myriad of situations involving returns and credit situations. Exhibit 1-10 is a procedure that details the proper preparation and use of this form, and so should be studied in order to understand the complexities that can arise.

One situation that should be addressed is the charge versus no-charge return. A charge return is one involving a credit to be received by the hospital. A no-charge return is one that involves return of "free" material. The mechanics of a charge return is the basis of Exhibit 1-10. The form is completed and distributed in accordance with the procedure. The question to be resolved is how the no-charge procedure is effected with the use of this form. The answer lies in how the material was brought into the hospital. If the material was ordered for evaluation on a purchase order, the return procedure is handled exactly the same as a charge

Exhibit 1-9 Return Material/Credit Memorandum

RETURN MATERIAL/CREDIT MEMORANDUM

ST. FRANCIS HOSPITAL
12935 South Gregory Street
Blue Island, Illinois 60406

RM _____

S
H
I
P

T
O

REASON FOR THIS MEMORANDUM			
☐ RETURN FOR CREDIT ONLY DO NOT RETURN OR REPLACE	☐ UNAUTHORIZED DELIVERY	☐ LOAN MATERIAL RETURNED	☐ OVERSHIPMENT
☐ DAMAGED	☐ RENTAL RETURN	☐ TRIAL MATERIAL RETURNED	☐ INVOICE CORRECTION
☐ MATERIALS RETURNED FOR NON-CONFORMANCE WITH SPECIFICATIONS	☐ PICK UP MATERIAL	☐ SAMPLES RETURNED	☐ OTHER _____

DATE	DATE SHIPPED	SHIPPED VIA	RETURN	VENDOR'S INVOICE NO.	PURCHASE ORDER NO.	DEPARTMENT
			☐ PREPAID ☐ COLLECT			

ITEM NO.	QUANTITY / UNIT	DESCRIPTION	CODING DEPT.	CODING ACCT.	PRICE PER UNIT	AMOUNT
					TOTAL	$

BY _____

Exhibit 1-10 Return Material/Credit Memorandum Procedure

```
                                            PROCEDURE
                                            MMPD-009


                    ST. FRANCIS HOSPITAL
                    BLUE ISLAND, ILLINOIS


                 MATERIEL MANAGEMENT DEPARTMENT
                 PURCHASING DIVISION

                 RETURN MATERIAL/CREDIT MEMORANDUM

                          POLICY

    Any material returned or credit due the hospital must be
    supported by a Return Material/Credit Memorandum.

                          PURPOSE

    To provide the necessary supportive documentation.

                         PROCEDURE

    I. Definitions

    A. Return for Credit Only. Do Not Return or Replace.  Use of
    this item is for the express purpose of receiving credit from
    the vendor.

         Actions: Vendor: issues pickup order and credit memo.

                  Accounting:  withhold payment on specified invoice
                  pending receipt of credit from vendor.

    B. Damaged.  Used to inform vendor of a return for reason stated.

         Actions:  Vendor: 1. when used in conjunction with "A"
                   above, vendor is expected to issue a credit;
                   2. when used alone, vendor is expected to (a)
                   arrange for pickup of damaged item(s) and issue
                   credit memo; and (b) reship and rebill for
                   replacement merchandise.

    C. Material Returned For Non-conformance with Specification.
    Used when an unauthorized substitute is received or material
    received that does not conform with hospital specification.

         Actions: Vendor: 1. when used in conjunction with "A" above,
                  vendor is expected to issue credit; 2. when used
                  alone, vendor is expected to (a) reship and rebill
                  for correct item; and (b) issue credit for original
                  item(s) shipped.

    D. Unauthorized Delivery.  Used to return material which was
    not ordered by the hospital.

         Actions: Same as those listed in "A" above.
```

Exhibit 1-10 continued

```
                                              PROCEDURE
                                              MMPD-009
                                              Page 2.
```

E. Rental Return. Used to establish documentation for return
and exact dates of use.

    Actions: Vendor: arranges for pickup and issues billing
             billing for rental period.
             Accounting: uses form to verify rental period
             and confirm invoice.

F. Pickup Material. Used to identify that vendor is responsible
to arrange for pickup of material returned for another reason
indicated on form.

G. Loan Material Returned. Used to confirm return of material
borrowed for temporary use.

H. Trial Material Returned. Used to confirm return of material
used for evaluation. Must be used with "A".

I. Samples Returned. Used to confirm return of samples to
vendor.

J. Overshipment. Used to return overshipment of material to
vendor. Must be used with "A".

    Actions: Same as "A" above.

K. Invoice Correction. Used to identify need for vendor to
issue a credit for incorrect billing.

II. Completion of Form.

A. RM _____ - enter control number of this form. Forms will
        be consecutively numbered during the calander year, i.e.,
        80-001.

B. Upper Left Hand Corner - enter vendor name and address.

C. Ship To - enter vendor address if different from upper left
        hand corner.

D. Reason For This Memorandum - place an "X" in the appropriate
        box or boxes.

E. Date - enter date form is originated

F. Date Shipped - enter date material is to be returned.

G. Shipped Via - enter mode of shipment used.

H. Return - check either prepaid or collect.

I. Vendor's Invoice No. - enter the appropriate invoice number

J. Purchase Order Number - enter hospital purchase order number.

K. Department - enter name of department affected by this
        transaction.

Exhibit 1-10 continued

L. Item No. - enter item number from original purchase order
   of item affected.

M. Quantity/Unit - enter total quantity and unit of measure
   affected by this transaction.

N. Description - enter complete description of the material.

O. Coding - enter department number of affected department.

    Acct. Enter proper account affected by this transaction.

P. Price Per Unit - enter price per unit for which credit is
   expected. If non-charge item enter N/C.

Q. Amount - enter extended amount of anticipated credit
   (Qty X unit Price). If non-charge item enter N/C.

R. Total - enter total amount of credit for all items listed
   on this form.

S. By - enter signature of individual initiating this form.

III. Distribution of Form.

    A. Original - to vendor (serves as packing slip)

    B. Second copy - to accounting

    C. Third Copy - to receiving

    D. Fourth Copy - maintained by purchasing with original
       purchase order.

Director, Materiel Management

procedure. The form is marked N/C for no-charge in the unit price and amount columns. For material brought into the hospital when a purchase order was not utilized—for example, samples—the form is completed to provide documentation of the return to the vendor. Again, the symbol N/C is used to denote no-charge. Distribution of the form may be limited to purchasing, receiving, and the vendor. Accounting would not be sent a copy because no financial implications are involved in the transaction.

SUMMARY

The purchasing system is the basis of any successful purchasing program. Examples of form design and content have been provided here for inspiration, and to enable the practitioner to apply them to the needs of a particular hospital. The design of all forms should be compatible with the purchase order, and yet distinctive enough to provide form identity and recognition. Design, however, is secondary to content. The content of each form must contain the necessary elements for a legal contract. Although certainly other ideas do exist in relation to use, design, and content, the basics still remain of the utmost importance in documenting and organizing any hospital purchase.

NOTE

1. Uniform Commercial Code, sec. 2-201. Found in Ronald A. Anderson and Walter A. Kumpf, *Business Law,* 9th ed. (Cincinnati, Ohio: South-Western Publishing Co., 1973).

Chapter 2

Proper Purchasing Equals Quality

The first criterion in the purchasing process is quality determination. Like a rare, beautiful butterfly, its illusiveness can frustrate every attempt at capture. Yet, you persist until your desire has been fulfilled. Many times fulfillment requires the use of a larger net and a change in strategy until the capture has been made. So it is with quality. In this chapter we explore the tools available to aid the practitioner in proper quality determination.

Quality can be defined as that characteristic, property, or attribute that makes or helps to make an item usable. Said another way, quality is a physical or individual property or attribute that distinguishes (raises to a higher level or superior position) one product from an apparently identical product required for a specific use or purpose.

Quality determination can be real or imaginary. For example, if you were to ask various members of the nursing staff why they preferred brand A 4 ×4 sponges to brand B, the response might be that brand A is superior in quality. And if you were to ask the basis for this opinion, you might hear something akin to: "I have used it for so long, I know it has superior quality!" Real or imaginary?

For the practitioner, quality determination must be based on an objective (real) rather than subjective (imaginary) approach. The first step in an objective analysis is to define the function the product is to perform or accomplish. Defining the function of the product is the responsibility of the user and is usually first stated in general terms, for example, "something with which to sharpen pencils."

Once the basic function has been defined, other elements of the product's physical makeup enter the process of refining the quality determination. Some of the elements that influence quality determination include, but are not limited to, composition, color, durability, efficiency of operation, operating and service requirements, size, suitability, and technique of use. Each of these elements has its place in objectively analyzing any given product. Since every product must be judged upon its own merits, some of the elements will be weighted more heavily

27

than others; some will apply and some will not. Returning to the pencil sharpener example, one can begin to refine and define the desired quality. If the functional terminology of "something with which to sharpen pencils" is applied in general terms, a simple pocketknife could be utilized to meet the functional requirement of sharpening pencils. However, a simple pocketknife is probably not what the user had in mind. Refining our pencil sharpener requirements will require some necessary questions to acquire a more accurate definition of what the user is seeking. Typically, these questions would include:

- Is the unit manual or electric?
- If manual, must it be wall mounted or does it require a vacuum base?
- Will the unit be required to sharpen standard or multisized pencils?
- How large a receptable is needed?
- What color should the unit be?

There are other questions that can apply in seeking the proper definition of our pencil sharpener requirements. The important point is that these types of questions can and should be utilized in defining the functional quality requirements for any given product.

Quality determination is a responsibility that cannot be placed on the practitioner alone. User participation is a necessity from a purely technical perspective. In today's rapidly changing technological climate, no practitioner can be expected to know everything there is to know about every product that is purchased for use within the hospital. The purchasing practitioner's role is to seek out new products and services and present the information to the user for evaluation.

It is also the practitioner's role to ensure that every product or service receives a thorough and fair evaluation. The evaluation process can be accomplished through the use of pilot studies, a panel of experts, and specification development, to name a few methods. Pilot studies involve the selection of one or more user departments that will use the product for a specified time period. At the end of the evaluation period, all of the personnel involved complete a questionnaire prepared especially for the evaluation.

The use of experts requires the selection of personnel familiar with the type of product in question. The experts utilize comparative testing and qualitative analysis to determine if the product meets the established criteria for performance, effectiveness, quality, and safety. On the basis of the results of the testing, the experts recommend approval or rejection of the product.

Specification development, as a quality determination technique, is explored in greater detail later in this chapter.

There will also be times when, in order to ensure the effectiveness of an evaluation, the practitioner will be required to play the role of "devil's advocate." The role often requires the asking of some difficult questions of the user in order to ensure fairness. The role should be assumed only in those situations where the user may be "blowing smoke" to cover up the real reason(s) for not accepting any given product. Practitioners must also remember that the answer to the acceptability of the technical quality of any product rests with the user.

VALUE ANALYSIS

Value analysis is one of the most objective techniques available to aid in quality determination. Defined, value analysis is an investigative process that systematically studies every element of a material, component, or service in terms of its function and its associated cost to develop the most effective quality specification at the most cost-effective price. Value analysis is a problem-solving approach that challenges the use and specification of, and the need for, any given product or service.

Before we consider the technique employed with value analysis, it is important to look at the word "value." Value is a word that can be expressed in terms of use, cost, esteem, or exchange.

Use value is based on the elements and qualities of any given material or service in relation to the purpose of that material or service. Use value is normally objective.

Cost value, as one would suspect, is based upon the cost of a product or service and is normally expressed monetarily.

Esteem value is based upon the attractiveness involved through ownership of the item or use of a particular service and is subjective.

Exchange value is based upon the elements or qualities that make an item exchangeable for something else.

These four types of value are presented to emphasize that the primary concerns of value analysis are of use and cost values. Esteem and exchange values have no place in the use of value analysis. For any item or service to achieve high value, emphasis should be placed on obtaining the highest use value at the most cost-effective price.

Value analysis is applied by subjecting the item or service to a series of questions. The opportunity for cost reduction may exist if an item fails any of the questions.

1. Does the use of the item contribute value? This question seeks to determine whether a useful and necessary purpose exists for the item or service. The answer should clearly state the function(s) the user requires.

2. Is its cost proportionate to its usefulness? Based upon the desired function, the question seeks to determine whether a lower cost item will accomplish the same function.
3. Does the item need all of its features? This question seeks to eliminate all of the unnecessary bells and whistles manufacturers add to enhance an item.
4. Is there anything better for the intended use? This question is directed not at the lowest priced product, but to the product that performs the desired function most efficiently and economically.
5. Can a standard product be found that will be usable? This question is meant to force a review of current products already in use that may be able to perform the desired function (see section on standardization).
6. Can the product or service be accomplished in-house for less? This question raises the issue of evaluating buying versus making a given product or service utilizing underutilized resources already available in the hospital.
7. Will another dependable supplier provide it for less? This is a purchasing function that is accomplished through competitive bidding and negotiation.
8. Is anyone buying it for less? Again, this is a purchasing function that can be accomplished by surveying other hospitals and/or businesses currently using the product or service.

STANDARDIZATION

As noted in question 5, standardization is a proper part of value analysis. One of the problems the practitioner may encounter in establishing a standardization program is the "indifference to standardization" syndrome. This syndrome is characterized by the preference for certain brands without regard for quality or cost. Indifference to standardization is like a cancer; left unchecked it will consume the whole and result in chaos for purchasing.

Every hospital should have a standardization program that promotes simplification; reduction in the number of types, sizes, etc., in inventory; and elimination of the extra procedures necessary to purchase special items.

Establishing a good standardization program requires the following actions by the practitioner.

For inventory items:

1. Analyze current inventory to identify duplications.
2. Review annual usage and inventory carrying costs to determine total annual costs for the hospital.
3. Present your findings to the users as a group to facilitate the decision-making process. Utilize qualitative value analysis.

For noninventory items:

1. Analyze purchases by department or commodity for duplication (e.g., orthopedic soft goods used by surgery, physical therapy, emergency room).
2. Present items to users (medical staff committees or department heads) for decision-making process.

Other actions:

1. Get out from behind your desk and establish contact with the departments and medical staff. Become a promoter and get out and sell your product, standardization.
2. Discontinue purchasing products on the basis of a few brands; give consideration to the products of all companies.
3. Coordinate buying and reduce the variety of the items purchased.
4. Establish standards or definitions of quality that will make it possible to obtain competitive bids on items purchased in large quantities.
5. Require that products conform to the established standard. Make it a practice never to accept substitutes without prior approval.

Sounds simple doesn't it? Well, do not be lulled into complacency. Standardization requires diligence, assertiveness, and persistence. Remember, indifference is like a cancer. Simply trying to "cut it out" does not alway ensure success. Preventive medicine, accomplished through continued checkups, is a necessary component of a successful program.

THE STANDARDS COMMITTEE

The most popular technique used by hospitals to resolve the problems associated with product evaluation and standardization has been the standards committee. Employed correctly, the use of a committee approach to organized evaluation and standardization can be one of the most effective methods available to the purchasing practitioner and the user departments.

From a review of virtually every publication written on standards committees, two facts have become apparent. The first is that Charles Housley has undoubtedly proposed the most complete, idealized dissertation on this subject that has ever been written.[1] Housley's concept of the standards committee is something each practitioner should establish as a model and a goal to be reached.

The second fact is that other authors offer unique, innovative approaches that have worked well for them. The common thread that binds them together is that each committee has been developed according to the individual hospital's political environment. Political environment, as it is used here, refers to the organized structure of the hospital, and the personalities involved in directing or influencing the direction of the organization. Certain individuals or groups (other than administration), because of their strong personalities or positions, will exert greater influence than perhaps they should. As proposed by Housley and other authors, the standards committee can become one of the strongest political groups in the hospital. For this reason, the purchasing practitioner should approach the organization or reorganization of the standards committee from the viewpoint of what can realistically be accomplished, given the political environment of the hospital. Ideally, it would be wonderful if the practitioner did not have to be concerned with political environment. However, politics exists in every organization and is, by necessity, a consideration that must be dealt with. In the truest sense, this is the wisdom of reality. Thus, the practitioner will need to tailor the concept of the standards committee to the political climate of the hospital. With this "tailor-made" concept as a basis, the practitioner should use the following as a guide to organizing or reorganizing the standards committee.

The practitioner should begin by defining the role of the committee. As previously noted, evaluation and standardization are by-products of value analysis. Thus, the committee's primary role should be to analyze products to determine their effectiveness in meeting the operational requirements necessary to meet, in turn, the needs of the patient or the hospital.

Once the role of the committee has been defined, the next requirement is to obtain the necessary decision-making authority from administration. The standards committee should be responsible for ensuring the proper testing and evaluation of all products that lie within its sphere of authority. Ideally, the standards committee should be the final decision-making authority for all supplies and noncapital equipment used in the hospital. As a practical matter, the authority of the committee should also be approved by the medical staff. Support of the medical staff is imperative if the committee is to be an effective, functional entity in the hospital.

Committee membership should include representatives from both clinical and nonclinical departments. A suggested core group would include representatives from administration, accounting, clinical engineering, infection control, nursing, materiel management/purchasing, and medical staff. This core group, supplemented by department heads who request product analysis, should be sufficient to facilitate the decision-making process. Committee appointments should be made by the administrator.

Requests for product review should follow a definite standard procedure. Whenever possible, products should be recommended by a department director and reviewed by the clinical committee related to the specific area, if one exists. For example, the pediatrics committee of the medical staff would review products relating to the nursery and pediatrics departments. This type of review process tends to accomplish three things: (1) It provides for specialized clinical review and comment prior to presentation to the standards committee. (2) Poor or unworkable recommendations are "weeded out." (3) Where specific products are unknown, it tends to promote finalization of function and specification. For products recommended to the standards committee, the individual who initiated the request or the department head should be invited to participate in the committee discussion. This participation by the requesting department tends to create a positive environment.

The use of an agenda is a necessity. The agenda should be sent out along with copies of the necessary documentation relating to agenda items. As the chairperson, the practitioner must keep the meetings running as smoothly as possible. One of the problems generally associated with committees in general is that the members would prefer to be somewhere else. The bywords here are productivity and a sense of accomplishment.

The final point is to measure the effectiveness of the committee. Other authors believe the committee's effectiveness should be measured quantitatively in terms of the dollars saved. This author disagrees. The true effectiveness of a committee cannot be measured in dollars and cents alone. Effectiveness is using or manipulating the political environment in favor of prudent use of the hospital's resources and improvement of the quality of patient care. After all, isn't quality patient care the overall objective of a hospital?

WRITING A SPECIFICATION

Once all of the elements of acceptable quality have been determined, the next step is to establish a product specification to provide the vendors with a clear understanding of what the hospital is looking for, as well as a basis for inspection following delivery. Normally, although a quality specification cannot be written out in detail on every purchase order or agreement, it is a necessary part of every purchase agreement. Quality specifications, therefore, are generally utilized in competitive bidding procedures to determine which product or group of products will meet the hospital's requirements. Within the hospital industry, quality specifications are generally expressed by the use of one or more of the following: hospital-developed purchase specification, brand name, catalog designation, and market grade.

Purchase Specification

Hospital-developed specifications are perhaps the least used of all the methods for expressing the quality requirements of the hospital. The principal reason for this lack of use is that the practitioner assumes the responsibility to describe the hospital's requirements in complete, positive terms. Many practitioners feel they are unable to perform this function adequately, and rightfully so. Development of a purchase specification is the responsibility of the user, not the practitioner.

Practitioners who intend to write their own specifications for quality determination require a few words of caution. Writing purchase specifications for every item purchased may not be economical because of the cost of preparation; for example, for small, nonrepetitive purchases, of which there are many. It must also be recognized that the practitioner assumes the responsibility for the performance of a product, since the practitioner has determined its composition, and possibly the method of manufacture. The practitioner should be very familiar with the product or service being specified, not only as a basis for preparing clear, concise specifications, but also to prevent the hospital from incurring additional expenses as a result of poor performance. Therefore, it is more important that the practitioner use the various methods of quality specification wisely than to be able to prepare purchase specifications for every item purchased for use within the hospital.

For practitioners who will utilize purchase specifications as one method of expressing the quality requirements of the hospital, the following methodology and explanations are provided. Purchase specifications must not be written so restrictively that the number of potential vendors limits the availability of competition. The specifications should be broad enough to provide an equal opportunity to all qualified vendors, and yet stringent enough to ensure the maintaining of high quality standards while excluding products that may be undesirable from a quality perspective. A well-written specification will inform the vendors clearly and concisely of the characteristics that must be included in the product or service to produce the results desired by the hospital. Well-written specifications will also serve as evidence that careful thought has been given to the intended use of, need for, and specific characteristics of the items that are demanded to satisfy the need.

Purchase specifications normally will contain any or all of four key elements: composition, physical dimensions or measurements, performance, and method of manufacture. Exhibit 2-1 is a purchase specification that employs some of the key elements on at least a limited scale. The requirements for polished stainless steel provide the element of composition. The size definition provides the element of physical dimension, although a scale drawing, if included, would more clearly define the physical dimensions. Line 5 provides the concept of manufacture "welded by heli-arc method." Only the element of expected performance has not been included.

Exhibit 2-2 provides a more accurate description of the element of performance. This excerpt from a specification for microfilm services clearly places a burden on the vendor to supply a brand of film and a process that will meet the needs of the hospital.

As previously noted, purchase specifications are expensive to prepare and should be used wisely. Capital equipment and repetitive high-dollar-volume items are probably worth the effort involved. Any system of purchase specifica-

Exhibit 2-1 Purchase Specification—Kick Bucket

ST. FRANCIS HOSPITAL
BLUE ISLAND, ILLINOIS

PURCHASE SPECIFICATION

Product: Kick Bucket, Stainless Steel

Specification:

1. Size: 14½-inch diameter, 12⅝ inches high;
2. Polished stainless steel, nonmagnetic, 18-8G;
3. Base and uprights 12G polished stainless steel;
4. Channel and pail 16G polished stainless steel;
5. Welded by heli-arc method;
6. Four (4) "L" shaped uprights, 1½ inches wide, welded to top of carrier base, continuous conductive rubber bumper set into channel and entire unit mounted on four (4) ball bearing swivel casters, 2 inches, with conductive rubber wheels;
7. Seamless 12-quart pail

Primary User(s): Emergency Room, Surgery

Prepared By: _____

Date Prepared: _____
Review Dates:

Exhibit 2-2 Purchase Specification—Microfilm

B. MICROFILM PROCEDURE - ROLL FILM

  1. The film used will be high resolution permanent
      type microfilm. The processed microfilm will
      contain a triangle in the margin indication that
      the film meets Federal Standards for permanence,
      as specified in American National Standards PH 1.28.

  2. All processed microfilm will contain less than 0.005
      milligrams per square inch of residual ammonium
      or sodium thiosulfate (hypo), and will meet American
      National Standard PH 4.8 for archival permanence.

  3. Each film roll shall contain not less than 18 inches
      of film leader and 18 inches of film trailer. It
      is understood that the hospital will, at its option,
      take film rolls at random and submit short strips
      of film, taken from the leader or trailer, to an
      independent laboratory for testing as per (a) above.

  4. The background density of the processed microfilm
      images shall be not less than 0.9 nor more than 1.3
      difuse transmission density. This measurement will
      be made in accordance with American National Standards
      PH 2.17 and PH 2.19.

  5. The resolution of the completed microfilm shall be
      not less than 80 lines per millimeter as determined
      by using National Bureau of Standards Microcopy Test
      Chart No. 1010a. Resolution is the result of high
      quality cameras, lens, and film. The camera must be
      in proper adjustment and high quality processing are
      also required.

tions requires updating, a process that should reflect the combined effort of purchasing and the user. User involvement should be encouraged. The resourceful and imaginative practitioner will soon discover that the time spent on preparation and user involvement will result in leading the user away from brand name purchasing.

Brand Name

An alternative to the detailed purchase specification is the use of a recognized brand name. Brand name specification is simple and offers some advantages over purchase specifications. These include:

- Vendors more readily understand the hospital's requirements.

- User acceptance is more readily obtained.

- Practitioners can be assured of obtaining the desired product.

One disadvantage of using brand names is that it effectively eliminates competition at the manufacturer's level. And one way to overcome this disadvantage is the use of an "acceptable brand names" list, which names manufacturers whose products have been accepted as meeting the required quality or performance standards of the hospital. Use of a brand names list is particularly effective in construction programs, and when products from a number of manufacturers will meet the hospital's requirements adequately.

Catalog Description

The use of catalog numbers or descriptions is closely associated with brand name specification. While the desired quality is easily recognizable to the vendor whose catalog is used, it may prohibit competition by other vendors. Catalog descriptions can be effectively utilized provided the practitioner converts the description from the specific to the generic, by eliminating or modifying descriptions of components or features that are applicable to only one manufacturer. Such conversions usually can be facilitated by comparing all of the catalog descriptions for the various manufacturers and extracting the most common and necessary features or components. Although preparation of this type of specification is time consuming, the practitioner may prefer this method to a brand names list.

A word of caution relative to the use of catalog descriptions and brand name specification is necessary. The addition of the phrase "or equal" to a catalog number or brand name for bidding purposes is generally considered unsatisfactory. The term "or equal" is not clear or concise, and leaves the quality determination to the vendor Listing all of the acceptable manufacturers and their associated product numbers is a much better way to communicate desired quality.

Market Grade

As a method of quality specification, market grade is highly accepted and is most often used in the purchase of food commodity items. Market grades are normally established by government agencies, trade associations, or commodity authorities. Use of market grades for some commodities is one method of establishing quality standards. However, at best, market grades are generalizations that may allow for some fluctuation in quality.

QUALITY ASSURANCE

Regardless of what method is used to describe quality, a regular program should be established to ensure that the quality specified is being maintained by the manufacturer and/or vendor. At times, product manufacturing methods or specifications are modified without the hospital's knowledge. Thus, an inspection program should be undertaken to examine the product periodically for desired quality.

PRICE VERSUS COST ANALYSIS

For the purchasing practitioner, the ability to distinguish between price and cost and to perform a price/cost analysis are necessary skills. Most hospitals have personnel in the accounting department who can perform this function, but every practitioner should be familiar with the fundamental processes involved.

Price analysis is achieved by subjecting two or more comparable items to an analysis of their respective direct costs. This can be as simple as comparing the purchase costs of Kendall versus Johnson & Johnson 4× 4 gauze sponges, or as complex as Exhibit 2-3 for copy machines.

Cost analysis, on the other hand, encompasses all of the factors involved in the procurement, use, and disposal of any given product. Price analysis is but one factor in the cost analysis formula. Cost analysis seeks to quantify all of the expenses, such as transportation, receiving, handling, recording, and storage, which must be added to the price to determine the ultimate costs. Of the two analytical techniques, cost analysis provides a more complete picture of true expense. (See Exhibit 2-4 for an example of a cost analysis document.)

Exhibit 2-3 Price Analysis

```
                    HOSPITAL PRICE ANALYSIS

                         COPY MACHINES

OBJECTIVE:   This analysis is to provide a cost comparison
             between two competitive copy machines.

GENERAL INFORMATION

The analysis is based upon information provided by the
respective manufacturers.  Both units are comparable in
respect to features offered and copy quality.  Supply
costs are based upon best quantity purchases.  Copier "B"
is currently in use.

DATA BASE

      Estimated copies per month:  24,000

      Term of Contract:  2 years

      Paper Costs:  $3.25/ream or 0.0065 each

COMPARISON

1.  Copier A

      Monthly Rental                          $180.00

         Copies included in rental:  6,000

         Additional cost per copy:  $0.01 up to 26,000

Monthly Copies               24,000

Less copies included          6,000
                             18,000 x $0.01         $180.00

Toner:  20.29 fluid ounces @ $20.00 ea
        1 bottle = 12,000 copies $20.00 x 2 ea      $ 40.00

Dispersant:  32 oz. bottle @ $2.00 ea
        1 bottle = 8,000 copies $2.00 x 3 ea        $  6.00

Paper Costs:  24,000 = 48 reams x $3.25             $156.00
                500

Total Monthly Cost                                  $562.00

Cost per copy:  $562.00 = $0.023 each
                24,000 copies
```

Exhibit 2-3 continued

```
Price Analysis
Copy Machines
Page 2


2.  Copier B

    Monthly Rental                                          $ 415.00

    Copies included in rental:  8,750

    Additional Cost per copy:

        8,750 to 20,000 = $0.0205

        20,000 plus      = $0.016

    Monthly copies        24,000

    Less copies included  8,750
                          15,250  x $0.0205        $ 312.625

    Toner:  6 oz. bottle @ $6.125
            1 bottle = 5,000 copies $6.125 x 4.8 ea $  29.40

    Dispersant:  32 oz. bottle @ $8.40
            1 bottle - 10,000 copies $8.40 x 2.4 ea $  20.16

    Paper costs:   24,000  = 48 reams x $3.25     $ 156.00
                   ------
                     500

    Total Monthly Cost                            $ 933.185

    Cost per copy:  $933.185   = $0.039 each
                    24,000 copies


SUMMARY

Monthly operating costs of Copier A      $562.00
Annual Costs:    $562.00 x 12 months                 $ 6,744.00

Monthly operating costs of Copier B      $933.185
Annual Costs:    $933.185 x 12 months                $11,198.22

Copier A affords annual cost savings of $ 4,454.22 over
Copier B.
```

Exhibit 2-4 Cost Analysis

```
                    HOSPITAL COST ANALYSIS

                    MICROFILM SERVICES


OBJECTIVE:   This analysis is to provide a cost comparison for
             a decision on using a service company versus an
             in-house microfilm program.


GENERAL INFORMATION

With the exception of Medical Records, no microfilming has
ever been accomplished at the hospital.  The desire to have a
microfilming program has been discussed over the last several
years with no definitive action being taken.

At the present time, there are a number of departments
utilizing record storage space that has been made available
in another building.  This storage space is in a chaotic
state, exceeding its designed capacity.

The Medical Reocrds Department is the only department that
has ever had records filmed.  All medical records prior to
1957 have been microfilmed using a roll film format.  All
inactive records from 1957 to 1968 are currently maintained
in a storage area one floor below the department.  The primary
storage area within Medical Records is current beyond capacity
to the point where the actual floor load may exceed design
capacity.  This area has the most critical need for a micro-
filming program.

Other departments including:  Laboratory, Payroll, Cardiology,
Nuclear Medicine, Accounting, Business Office, and Personnel,
are now or shortly will be in need of a microfilm program
due to limited record storage space.

A detailed record survey of the affected departments yielded
the following data.

Medical Records:  Years 1957-1968, 95,588 records averaging
      51 images per reocrd equalled 4,875,000 total images.

      Years 1969-1971, 11,410 records averaging 195 images
      per record equalled 2,225,000 total images.

Business Office:

   Inpatient Records 1976 - 1978, 49,970 records averaging
   30 images per record equalled 1,482,000 total images.

   Outpatient Records 1976 - 1978, 159,672 records averaging
   8 images per record equalled 1,277,000 total images.
```

Exhibit 2-4 continued

```
Cost Analysis
Microfilm Services
Page 2


    Income Daily Summary Reports 1976 - 1978, 300 reports per
    year averaging 290 images per report equalled 261,000
    total images.

Accounting Department:  1974 - 1977 Payables vouchers, 40,000
    vouchers averaging 10 images per voucher equalled 400,000
    total images.

Payroll Department:  1974-1977 70,200 Time Cards averaging
    2 images per card equalled 140,400 total images.

Personnel Department:  1800 personnel records averaging 10
    images per record equalled 18,000 total images.

Laboratory:  1976 - 1978 25,000 lab reports equalled 25,000
    total images.

ECG:  1977 - 1979 patient records, 22,000 records per year
    averaging 7 images per record equalled 300,000 total
    images.

Nuclear Medicine:  1976 - 1979 11,500 records per year averaging
    3 images per record equalled 104,000 images.


TOTAL IMAGES ALL DEPARTMENTS  9,625,400

Service Company Costs:  The below listed costs are based upon
acceptance of the low bid.  All bids were based upon the pre-
viously listed image totals.

    Medical Records
        Records for years 1957 - 1968          $ 44,884.00
        Records for years 1969 - 197]          $ 38,381.00

    Business Office
        Inpatient Records                      $ 25,875.00
        Outpatient Records                     $ 24,840.00
        Income Daily Summary Reports           $  3,761.00

    Accounting Department                      $  6,900.00
    Payroll Department                         $  2,421.00
    Personnel Department                       $    397.00
    Laboratory Department                      $    430.00
    ECG Department                             $  5,175.00
    Nuclear Medicine Department                $  1,795.00

                    TOTAL COST                 $154,859.00


In-House Program:  Because this program is to film limited
access records, roll filming will be assumed for all records.
```

Exhibit 2-4 continued

Cost Analysis
Microfilm Services
Page 3

1. Images per roll: Lens reduction ratio of 28:1. Feed
    length of average document is 11 inches plus 1/2 inch for
    space between documents for a total of 11 1/2 inches.

$$\text{Image Length} = \frac{11.5}{28} = 0.41$$

$$\text{Images/100 ft. roll} = \frac{1200 \text{ inches}}{0.41} = 2926 \text{ images}$$

2. Number of rolls required:

$$\frac{9,625,400 \text{ total images}}{2,926 \text{ images/roll}} = 3,290 \text{ rolls}$$

3. Film Costs: 3,290 rolls x $0.41/roll = $25,004.00

4. Film Processing: 3,290 rolls x $0.41/roll = $1,348.90

5. Preparation Costs: Assume labor rate of $5.20 per hour
    (includes all benefits). A sample run would be necessary
    for each type of document to find the actual cost of
    preparation. Staples must be removed and records
    arranged in standard sequence.

    Assume preparation of 4,000 documents per hour.

$$\frac{9,625,400}{4,000} = 2,406 \text{ hours x } \$5.30/\text{hr.} = \$12,751.80$$

6. Filming Costs: A rotary camera can film at a rate of 4,000
    images per hour. Because of fatigue factor (10%), we will
    assume 3,600 images/hour.

$$\frac{9,625,400}{3,600} = 2,674 \text{ hours x } \$5.30/\text{hr} = \$14,172.20$$

7. Inspection Costs: This will take approximately 15 minutes
    per roll or 0.25 hours.

    3,290 rolls x 0.25 = 822.5 hours x $5.30 = $4,359.25

8. Equipment Costs:

    1 ea Rotary Camera @ $7,569.00 $ 7,569.00

    1 ea Microfilm Processor @ $7,014.00 $ 7,014.00

    3 ea Chairs @ $150.00 $ 450.00

    2 ea Tables @ $150.00 $ 300.00

Exhibit 2-4 continued

```
Cost Analysis
Microfilm Services
Page 4


8.  Equipment Costs (continued):

    5 ea Reader/Printers @ $4,100.00          $20,500.00

    5 ea Readers @ $2,000.00                  $10,000.00

          Total Equipment Cash Cost          $45,833.00


    Depreciation based on straight line method for 5 years


      $45,833.00 = $9,166.60 equipment cost/year.
       5 years

9.  Room depreciation, lighting, heating and air conditioning
    costs are not included based upon use of an available room
    for which the costs are already computed within the budget.



Summary of Costs

    1.  In-House Program

        A.  Film Costs                        $ 25,004.00
        B.  Processing Costs                  $  1,348.90
        C.  Labor
              Preparation                     $ 12,751.80
              Filming                         $ 14,172.20
              Inspection                      $  4,359.25

        D.  Equipment (depreciated)           $  9,166.60
        E.  Equipment Service Contract        $    560.00
        F.  Paper Disposal (estimated)        $  3,000.00

                  Total                       $ 70,362.75

    2.  Service Company Costs

        A.  Filming                           $154,859.00
        B.  Readers & Reader/Printers
            depreciated                       $  6,100.00

                  Total                       $160,959.00


    3.  Cost Avoidance available through In-House Program

        $160,959.00 - $ 70,362.75 = $ 90,569.25
```

Before we review the actual process of cost analysis, three fundamental principles must be clarified. First, a *cost savings* results when the monies that would normally be spent are reduced. For example, if a hospital is spending $1000 per year for ballpoint pens and a reduction in the unit cost results in a reduction of total costs to $800, then a $200 cost savings has been achieved. Second, a *cost avoidance* results when available, underutilized resources are used instead of new or additional resources acquired. A cost avoidance also results when the wants and needs for a product are clarified and the wants (nice-to-have) features are eliminated—for example, assigning expediting duties to a clerk typist rather than hiring another individual to accomplish the expediting function.

And third, when dealing with an analysis that includes labor, a savings in labor costs occurs only when a position is eliminated from the budget. Improved efficiency resulting from a technological change without a budget reduction is not a savings. There must be an actual reduction in available budgeted hours to achieve a labor savings.

It is important that practitioners recognize the difference between a cost savings and a cost avoidance in order to understand and explain the results of any given cost study. It is also important that any labor savings achieved be just that, a savings. Failure to recognize these important points can result in poor information input into the decision-making process and could, ultimately, cause the hospital increased, unnecessary expenditures.

The first step in the cost analysis process requires that the objective or purpose for the cost analysis be stated clearly and concisely. For example:

• This analysis is to provide a cost comparison for a decision on using disposable diapers versus a diaper service.

• This analysis is to determine the cost of a Xerox copier versus an IBM copier.

• This analysis is to determine if the current charges for operating room disposables are reasonable and accurate.

Once the objective has been clearly stated, the second step is to determine what factors must be included to make an objective analysis. Typical factors influencing cost analysis include:

• supplies
• labor
• disposal problems
• inventory investment
• replacement costs

• capital investment
• maintenance costs
• depreciation costs
• alternative investment costs
• potential revenue

It is important to recognize that each cost analysis may require a different set of factors. What is applicable for one analysis may not be applicable for another analysis. The third step is to detail the source for each of the factors involved and the method of determination or computation. This detail work is necessary to provide documentation or "proof" of how the results were determined (see Exhibit 2-5). In a majority of cases, the cost analysis will be reviewed by the administrator, another department head, or the product utilization committee as part of the decision-making process. It is important that everyone involved in the decision understand how the results were arrived at (see Exhibit 2-6). No matter what the outcome of the analysis is, someone will challenge the final results. Therefore, the practitioner should be prepared to substantiate the methodology used (see Exhibit 2-7).

Finally, as a matter of routine, the practitioner should be prepared to follow up to ensure that a cost savings, cost avoidance, or increased revenue is realized. The analysis should be reviewed with the appropriate department head to determine whether the objective of the analysis has been accomplished.

As an aid to the reader, examples of a price analysis and a cost analysis are given in Exhibits 2-3 and 2-4. These examples are real. Your results may vary for similar studies. The results are less than important. The proper methodology is the important issue.

NOTE

1. Charles E. Housley, *Hospital Materiel Management* (Germantown, Md.: Aspen Systems Corp., 1978).

Exhibit 2-5 Sample Procedure

POLICY
MM-05

ST.FRANCIS HOSPITAL
BLUE ISLAND, ILLINOIS

MATERIEL MANAGEMENT DEPARTMENT

SUBJECT: Sole Source and Directed Purchases

OBJECTIVE:
To assure the proper development, approval, and documentation of all sole source and directed purchase requests in reference to supplies, equipment, and equipment services.

POLICY STATEMENT:
The Materiel Management Department will develop guidelines to purchase all supplies and equipment in accordance with the prudent buyer requirements of Sections 2102 and 2103 of the Provider Reimbursement Manual.

REFERENCED HOSPITAL POLICY:
To provide for optimal achievable care at a reasonable and justifiable cost.

DEFINITIONS:

Sole Source: Refers to purchase requests that indicate that the specified vendor is the only vendor that is acceptable to a department director or physician.

Directed Purchase: Refers to the selection of supplies, equipment, or equipment services by a department director or physician without consideration for established hospital standards and/or identical competitive materiel or service.

PROCEDURAL DOCUMENTATION:

1. Department directors or physicians are required to submit a letter to Materiel Management that provides specific documentation and justification why the request should not be subjected to established hospital standards, evaluation techniques, and/or competitive bidding.

2. All justifications must be reviewed and approved by Administration prior to a purchase order being issued.

3. For non-recurring purchases, Materiel Management will attach the justification letter to the associated purchase order.

4. For recurring purchases, Materiel Management will maintain the justification letter in the appropriate departmental file.

5. Letters of justification for recurring purchases must be updated by the department director or physician and approved by Administration annually.

EXCEPTIONS: None

Director, Materiel Management

Exhibit 2-6 Product Utilization Committee—Purpose and Policy

POLICY
PUC-001
5/1/81

ST. FRANCIS HOSPITAL
BLUE ISLAND, ILLINOIS

PRODUCT UTILIZATION COMMITTEE

PURPOSE

To monitor and control the use of supplies within the hospital with emphasis on the quality of care and the containment of costs.

POLICY

It shall be the policy of this hospital that any products which are proposed for use within the hospital must first undergo evaluation and approval by the Product Utilization Committee.

1.   All potential products (either for use or evaluation) must be submitted to the Product Utilization Committee by physicians, hospital personnel, sales representatives, etc.

2.   Value analysis will be applied to all product submittals as a basis for the decision making process.

3.   An agenda will be prepared and distributed at least one week prior to the next committee meeting.

4.   The committee shall meet at least monthly and also on an "as needed" basis.

5.   If the requesting department is not represented on the committee, then it may send one representative to present the item. This representative may vote in this one case.

6.   Possible committee actions are:
     A.   Acceptance of the product;
     B.   Non-acceptance of the product;
     C.   A 30 day evaluation;
     D.   A 60 day evaluation;
     E.   A 90 day evaluation.

7.   The products to be evaluated are to be paid for by the supplier, if at all possible. When this is not possible, the requesting department's budget will be charged for all necessary associated costs.

8.   Once an item has been reviewed and rejected, the product will not be reconsidered by the committee for at least one year, unless there is a favorable price or product change.

9.   If an item is approved, the requesting department is

Exhibit 2-6 continued

POLICY
PUC-001
Page 2
5/1/81

responsible for submitting a product orientation and utilization
procedure to the Product Utilization Committee for review before
the newly accepted product is actually purchased.

10.   The Chairman shall submit all newly proposed items to
Accounting for review and determination of patient charge (if
applicable) before the item is reviewed by the Product Utilization
Committee.

11.   The minutes of all committee meetings must be sent to the
Assistant Executive Director before any action is taken. If
the Assistant Executive Director does not approve of the stated
action or actions, this is communicated back to the committee
and the item or items are not purchased.

12.   When a product is approved as a replacement for an existing
product, all useable quantities of the old product will be used
prior to initiation of purchase of the new, replacement product.

COMMITTEE APPOINTMENTS

All committee appointments must be approved by the Executive
Director. Medical Staff appointment must be made by the
President of the Medical Staff.

EXCEPTIONS

All items must undergo the above procedure with two exceptions.
1.) If the product is requested on an emergency basis by a
physician, it can be purchased. However, this item and action
must be reviewed at the next committee meeting. 2.) Pharmaceuticals
and food items are exempt from this policy.

REVIEW

This procedure must be reviewed at least annually.

_____
Chairman

_____
Executive Director

_____
President, Medical Staff

Exhibit 2-7 Product Utilization Committee—Statement of Objectives and
Function

POLICY
PUC-002
5/1/81

ST. FRANCIS HOSPITAL
BLUE ISLAND, ILLINOIS

PRODUCT UTILIZATION COMMITTEE

STATEMENT OF OBJECTIVES AND FUNCTION

OBJECTIVES

1.   To provide the mechanism to insure an improved level of
patient care through product evaluation with emphasis on the
quality of care and the containment of costs.

2.   To evaluate the voluminous and continuous flow of new and
improved products.

3.   To reduce the expense of educating and training personnel
to many and varied products and techniques through standardization.

4.   To keep Administration, department directors, and medical
staff informed and abreast of changes in products.

5.   To assist department directors in understanding mutual
problems in reference to supplies.

6.   To minimize the quantities of inventory by reducing the
variety of products.

FUNCTION

1.   To provide a system for the introduction, review, and analysis
of products used within the hospital.

2.   To provide for the evaluation and selection of products
best suited to meet functional requirements for quality patient
care and departmental operations.

3.   To promote discipline in the selection of products aimed
at the upgrading of patient care and departmental efficiency.

4.   To promote the prudent use of the hospital's resources and
improvement of the quality of patient care.

_____
Chairman

_____
Executive Director

Chapter 3

Vendor Evaluations and Analysis Equal Service

The second criterion used in the purchasing decision-making process is service. How can service be defined? Is service simply getting your order processed and to your dock when you want it? Is it when the vendor representative responds to your "emergency" by picking up your order from the warehouse or borrowing from another hospital and delivering it to your office? Does the vendor provide good service by hiring and training only "qualified" representatives who know their product and do not waste your time? Is it service when the vendor representative details only quality products at low prices? Is it all or none of the above? Vendor service is all of these qualities, and *more*.

Since the beginning of time, purchasing practitioners have searched for the perfect vendor, one who consistently offers the highest quality products, lowest prices, best deliveries, and no back orders. Despite a valiant and courageous effort, the perfect vendor has yet to be found. The reason is simple. In the real world of hospital purchasing, the perfect vendor does not exist! What does exist is a large number of good ones, a few who are fair, and many who are considered poor. Vendor performance is a matter of what you want and what you are willing to accept.

MEASURING VENDOR PERFORMANCE

In their search for the perfect vendor, practitioners have devised measuring methods that range from geometric triangles to complicated ratings that measure everything from the representative's performance and the efficiency of the office staff to the courtesy of the truck driver. All of which is nonsense. The key to acquiring good vendor performance is communication between you and the vendor. A practitioner should not have to plead for good service. Good service is something to be demanded. But before you can demand good service, it is necessary to lay down the ground rules or standards to the vendor. See Exhibit 3-1 for one hospital's policy statement.

51

Exhibit 3-1 Hospital Policy Statement

SAINT FRANCIS HOSPITAL
12935 S. GREGORY ST.
BLUE ISLAND, ILLINOIS 60406
312/597-2000

WELCOME TO SAINT FRANCIS HOSPITAL

This information sheet is for the benefit of all Vendor Representatives, repairman, etc., who have or desire business at the Hospital. Observing the following rules, which are HOSPITAL POLICY, will promote better relations and should prevent embarrasing situations.

We prefer that persons coming into the Hospital on business wear some means of identification. Vendor representatives should not contact hospital personnel other than the Purchasing Manager, the Director of the Pharmacy, or the Director of the Dietary Department. When necessary to meet with other personnel, arrangements can be made with the Purchasing Manager.

INTERVIEW HOURS:

Purchasing Department Ex. 311	Tuesday, Wednesday, Thursday 9:00 A.M. to 11:00 A.M. 1:30 P.M. to 4:00 P.M.
Pharmacy Ex. 280	Monday thru Friday 8:00 A.M. to 12:00 Noon
Dietary Ex. 533	By Appointment Only

PURCHASE ORDERS

No order will be valid unless it bears a number and is signed by the Purchasing Manager. Verbal orders should not be accepted unless confirmed by an order number. We attempt to price all orders before they are placed and all purchases are governed by the conditions printed on the order.

NEW PRODUCTS

New products are submitted to the Standards and Evaluation Committee for review. If the committee believes the product worthy, the vendor will be requested to supply sufficient merchandise for a proper evaluation. A report, favorable or unfavorable, will be given to the vendor representative. He should not contact hospital personnel for evaluation replies.

Exhibit 3-1 continued

REPAIR SERVICE

Repair or Service personnel should register at the Purchasing Department office where an authorization badge will be issued. When the work is completed he should return to the Purchasing Department at which time a purchase order will be issued. A service ticket signed by the appropriate department supervisor and indicating the time in and time out must be submitted.

After 5:00 P.M. or during week-end periods, such personnel should report to the Information Desk in the Main Lobby for the authorization pass and to leave the service report. A purchase order will be assigned the next working day and the company will be notified.

SHIPMENTS AND DELIVERIES

Shipments should be made F.O.B. St. Francis Hospital on a prepaid basis. All packages should show the purchase order number and a packing slip must accompany each shipment. Deliveries should be made to our Receiving Department between the hours of 8:00 A.M. and 4:00 P.M., Monday through Friday. (Deliveries of necessary dietary products will be accepted on Saturday). Only small emergency orders, previously agreed to, will be accepted at the Information Desk after 4:30 P.M.

INVOICES

Invoices must be submitted in duplicate. After the receipt of the merchandise, discounted bills will be paid by the 10th of the following month and net bills by the 30th.

ETHICS

These regulations are necessary and are nothing more than good sound business practice. All of our personnel have been advised of these rules and we look for your support in maintaining them. Gifts or inducements offered to any employee by a business representative is forbidden and breach of this rule can lead to a discontinuation of business with the offending company.

The first standard is to provide a quality product. The need for a quality product is based upon the criteria and specifications developed through the evaluation and standardization process conducted by the hospital. Unless otherwise specified, substitutions should not be accepted from the vendor.

The second standard is that the vendor is expected to have a delivery performance of 95 percent or better on the first shipment. This standard applies only to those items that have been awarded to the vendor and are routinely ordered. Communication is a key to this standard. If the vendor has been provided with the anticipated volume, order frequency, and normal order quantity, this performance criterion can easily be met. This standard should not be applied to one-time order items because the vendor cannot possibly anticipate the need for these types of items.

This second standard can be measured objectively by dividing the number of line items completed on the first shipment by the number of line items ordered. As an example:

$$\frac{\text{Number of items completed}}{\text{Number of items ordered}} = \frac{19}{20} \times 100 = 95.0 \text{ percent}$$

Why should 95 percent be acceptable? Why not a higher number? There is nothing magical about a 95 percent fill rate. The number can be higher or lower, depending upon the level of performance desired by the individual practitioner. The important point is to provide a minimal achievement level for the vendor to reach. Once the minimum has been reached, the vendor should be encouraged to achieve the best and highest delivery performance possible. The future reward for such delivery performance should be the award of additional business by the hospital. Ninety-five percent is not an impossible figure to accomplish. It was chosen because it exemplifies excellence.

The frequency of this measurement is an individual decision. Normally, the top vendors should be checked routinely one month per quarter. The results of this routine check or "report card" should be discussed with the vendor. This sharing will accomplish two things: (1) show the vendor that you are serious about the standard; and (2) provide the opportunity to determine how the vendor's score can be improved.

The third vendor standard is to maintain a normal delivery time of seven days for all volume or routine purchases. With this standard the number of days elapsing between when the order is placed and when it is received is a variable. Rural areas may be subjected to a longer period, while metropolitan areas may have a shorter period. In either case, this standard can (and should) be negotiated with the vendor. The ability of the vendor to meet this standard will be highly dependent upon the timing and frequency of order placement by the practitioner.

The fourth standard is that the vendor is expected to provide a consistent pricing policy to the hospital. This standard is undoubtedly controversial and requires that the word "consistent" be defined. A consistent pricing policy is a policy that is compatible with the quality of the product and the service levels provided by the vendor. Consistent does not necessarily mean having the lowest price all of the time. What it does mean is having a fair price that is compatible with the first three hospital standards.

The realities of business require the vendor to make a profit. Profits are made through either higher prices or lower operating costs (i.e., inventory, freight, ordering costs, personnel, etc.). If the vendor is to meet the previous standards, it is imperative that the costs involved be recouped. The vendor has a right to receive a fair profit for the services provided. In return, the hospital should expect to pay a fair price for the service the vendor provides. It is a two-way street: you pay for what you get.

The fifth standard is providing an easy and efficient methodology for problem solving. The standard can be accomplished through frequent visits by the representative and/or by having a specific "customer service" person in the office. Experience has shown that the vendors who have one individual assigned as the office representative for specific accounts tend to be more effective than those who rely on a general office staff for this purpose. Whenever possible, it is highly recommended that practitioners get to know the "office" people either through occasional visits to the vendor or by having these people come to the hospital. The residual benefits from this type of personal contact will become apparent over the long term, with better understanding by both parties.

The sixth standard is the vendor's capacity to assist the hospital to achieve a reduction in processing costs in such areas as order processing, receiving, inventory carrying costs, and distribution. This standard is achieved through an analysis of how the vendor's order processing system interfaces with the hospital's order placement system and what other reactions are created because of the vendor's internal system. Realistically, any economies achieved by the hospital more than likely will result in economies by the vendor, thus creating a winning situation for both the hospital and the vendor.

These six standards should provide an adequate basis for vendor analysis and selection. The first, quality, is quantified by the hospital. The second and third can be measured objectively. The fourth, pricing, can be measured through competitive bidding or negotiation. The final two tend to be subjective by their very nature. Ideally, all practitioners would like to be able to make a purely quantitative measurement for vendor selection. As a practical matter, awarding business on the basis of service alone is not easy. Service is a factor that must be considered. Good service is the result of good communication and problem solving between you and the vendor. Remember, a low price isn't any good if you cannot get the merchandise when you need it.

BACKDOOR BUYING AND SELLING

Backdoor buying and selling are problems that every purchasing practitioner faces on a daily basis. Many practitioners feel that they lie strictly with the vendor representatives, but actually these problems are more complex and varied. They are an indication of some serious problems with the hospital's purchasing practices.

Backdoor Buying

Backdoor buying is as widespread and as serious as backdoor selling. In most cases, backdoor buying is initiated by hospital employees and is not limited to department managers and nursing supervisors. It extends from technicians to the administrator. The reasons for backdoor buying range from ignorance of hospital policy to lack of confidence in purchasing's ability to respond to the department's "special needs."

A written policy on hospital purchasing is worthless if it is not backed up by some type of action by the practitioner. Admittedly, it is difficult for a practitioner to insist on the prerogative when dealing with a higher department head or a member of administration. It requires tact and a persistent effort by the practitioner to oppose backdoor buying by these individuals. Short-term results should not be expected. Success will only come over the long term through discussions with the offending party.

A written policy is also worthless if not everyone is aware of the policy's existence. Employee turnover is something every business and hospital faces. New employees should be informed during their initial orientation of the written policy and the need for working with the purchasing department.

Another cause for backdoor buying is that the requisitioners express a lack of confidence in the practitioner's ability to respond to or understand their "special" needs. This problem is most often emotional on the part of the requisitioner. Its causes run the gamut from arrogance to overdependence on one individual vendor for technical assistance. Acceptance of this rationale will reduce the practitioner from a professional to a clerk who simply pushes paperwork. Combating the "special needs" problem is an arduous task. Patience and understanding are top requirements, but are secondary to listening. In order to resolve the problem, the practitioner must carefully search out the emotional cause. This can only be accomplished by listening to the offender's reasoning, sorting out the camouflage or smokescreen issues, determining the real issues, and working out a positive course of action. This is not an easy task. Nor is it one that can be learned by reading a book. It can come only through experience and human understanding.

Backdoor Selling

As a problem, backdoor selling also comes down to two causes. The first cause is vendor representatives who violate hospital policy. As with employees, this usually results from arrogance or lack of knowledge.

Arrogance on the part of the vendor representative is also an emotional issue resulting from a "bad" experience with the practitioner. A bad experience can range from the practitioner failing to follow up on a product left for evaluation to the representative believing that the practitioner cannot or does not want to understand the "technicalities" of a product. The realities of purchasing are that it is virtually impossible to know about, or even understand, all of the technical features of a given product or piece of equipment. Any representative who uses this tack is usually creating a smokescreen to cover some other problem, either a personality clash or a lack of self-confidence. Or the representative might just violate the policy because rules were made to be broken.

Lack of knowledge can be, and often is, the second cause for attempting backdoor selling. Vendors experience turnover with representatives that is usually greater than the personnel turnover in purchasing, as a department, or in the hospital as a whole.

As a cause, lack of knowledge can be resolved through communicating the hospital's policy on the representative's first visit to the purchasing department.

Closing the Backdoor

Closing the backdoor on buying and selling is not an impossible task. It is a task that requires diligence and deeds. The following are examples of actions that will help close the door.

- Work on improving communication with the users. Learn how to listen. All of us can hear, but only a few know how to listen.

- Try to improve your technical knowledge concerning the items you purchase. This can be accomplished by talking to the representatives, visiting plants, going to trade shows, and seminars, etc.

- Willingly accept and process tough requisitions, those where it is difficult to locate qualified suppliers.

- Process all requisitions as promptly as possible.

- Give credit to departments that have assisted purchasing (through proper procedure) in locating new sources of supply and cost savings.

- Use a system for getting information on new products to departments promptly, accurately, and completely.

- Establish a "tickler" file to follow up and obtain a department's evaluation of new products.

- Keep records on where backdoor buying and selling have resulted in poor quality, late delivery, excessive costs, or other inefficiencies.

- Develop a communication system to arrange all interviews through purchasing.

- Remind suppliers of the need to check with purchasing before visiting departments.

- Use a vendor pass system that requires signing in and out of purchasing.

- Insist that sample orders and trial materials be processed through receiving on a purchase order.

- Insist that product samples be left only with purchasing.

- Refuse to process invoices that do not have purchase order numbers.

- Publish a policy statement that includes administration and/or board of trustees approval.

These examples will aid in closing the backdoor. But it should be realized that the backdoor will never be completely closed and locked. Curbing backdoor buying and selling is like trying to teach children to close the door when coming into and going out of the house; it requires patience, constant reminding, and a firm hand.

THE VIEW FROM THE OTHER SIDE OF THE DESK

For every purchasing transaction that is consummated there are winners and losers. The vendor representative who is awarded the business feels that the hard work has paid off. As a practitioner, satisfaction comes from a good-quality product, good service, and a fair price. Everyone is happy, except the vendor representative who "lost" the business. He/she feels cheated and betrayed. Suddenly, you, the purchasing practitioner, have slipped from being a wonderful person to do business with to a "price conscious chiseler" who never gives anyone a break. Sound familiar? It should, because that is how many representatives feel about today's hospital purchasing practitioners.

Earlier in this chapter we looked at meeting the practitioner's wants and needs by the vendor. Well, vendors have wants and needs too. All too often, purchasing practitioners have not met those needs. What do the representatives want?

Discussions with vendor representatives reveal that they would like to see practitioners clearly define the ground rules on service and price. For example, vendors often welcome the fact that some objective measurement of service is being utilized. All they ask is that the measurement method be fair, objective, and equally applied, and that the methodology be explained to them. You, as a hospital employee, receive some type of evaluation as to how your supervisor perceives how good a job you are doing. You expect that evaluation to be fair, honest, and objective. Should the vendor expect less from you? If you make a mistake, you expect a second chance to redeem yourself. So does the vendor.

As for pricing, vendors want only a fair chance, which can be attained through competitive bidding and information sharing. Information sharing appears to be an area over which the losing vendor would like to cast a grey shadow. Many vendors will claim they did not have the same information as the winner did (the winner must have had some sort of advantage). One technique that can be used to counteract this claim is to have all of the prospective vendors meet at one time, receive the written bid requests, and ask any questions they may have. While some vendors may object to this procedure, it will certainly eliminate any claims relating to lack of information.

Vendors also complain about the lack of followthrough by purchasing. If a vendor provides samples of a new product, the vendor expects to receive an answer relative to its acceptability. Unfortunately, some vendors perceive that purchasing practitioners accept samples just to get rid of the representative. Many times, samples that are left with purchasing never find their way to users. Also, if samples are sent to the user, purchasing never follows up to gain the user's opinion "because I forgot about it." As a purchasing practitioner, you have a responsibility to both the vendor and the user. If you accept a sample, you accept the responsibilities that go with it; namely, to respond to the vendor.

Finally, vendor representatives expect practitioners to provide honest and straightforward answers. This applies equally to new products, service, pricing, and loss of business. Vendors do not expect to win every bid or to gain 100 percent of the hospital's business. Remember, in making the final decision, you have to have some specific reason(s) as a basis for the decision. There is nothing wrong with sharing this information with all vendors. In fact, vendor relationships tend to improve when vendors know what it will take on their part to get and keep the hospital's business. As a vendor representative recently related, "The representative's objective is to make money. Purchasing's objective is to save money. Through a common partnership, both objectives can be accomplished successfully."

Chapter 4

The Actual Purchase Equals Price

Of the three basic purchasing criteria—quality, service, and price—purchasing practitioners have been credited with being too "price conscious." Nevertheless, the price that is paid for an item is still a criterion that requires some type of decision making. For example, both the pressures for cost containment and the prudent buyer provision of Medicare law force the practitioner to deal with the issue of price.

COMPETITIVE BIDDING

Through competitive bidding, the hospital is afforded a wider choice of products and vendors. Since its objective is higher quality goods and services at lower prices, in theory this process should be applied to everything the hospital purchases. In the real world of hospital purchasing, however, this is not always possible, practical, or cost effective. Given the available time and the variety of commodities purchased by the hospital, competitive bidding should be used only where it results in the most value.

Why bid? There are three reasons for doing so. Competitive bidding should be used to:

1. spell out specifically what the hospital wants so the vendor can quote intelligently
2. provide the practitioner with all of the necessary facts on which to base a decision to place the order
3. furnish documentation of soliciting bids and reasons for making the award

What should be bid? As a routine, high volume A and B items should be competitively bid (see Chapter 10 for an explanation of ABC analysis). Because the dollars they represent are significant, these items require considerably more time and effort than low-dollar C items. As a general guide, supply items for which annual purchases total $500 or more should be competitively bid. Exhibit 4-1 is a sample policy. Commodity groups that, in the aggregate, represent a large volume should also be included in the bidding process. Capital equipment is a third area for competitive bidding. Finally, contract services, such as laundry processing, elevator maintenance, office machines, and medical equipment repair, should be subjected to competitive bidding as well.

Items covered by group purchasing agreements, emergency requests, single source items, and inventory C items are all areas where competitive bidding may not be advantageous.

Frequency

Bids should be solicited at least once a year, or just prior to the end of a price protection period. Annual bidding offers two advantages. First, it reduces the total time spent on processing routine reorders, thus freeing the practitioner to devote more time to problem solving and to processing nonrecurring purchases. And second, the vendor, provided with information as to the anticipated annual volume, can negotiate with manufacturers for better prices on the basis of improved volume purchasing, which will be passed on to the hospital. Further, it should also improve the vendor's inventory control procedures, and thus the vendor's ability to meet the hospital's routine demand cycle. Of course, the vendor should be given enough time to adjust inventory levels to meet the hospital's demand.

Procedure

Competitive bidding can be accomplished by using any of three basic techniques: telephone, representative visits, and formal written quotations.

The telephone represents a quick, convenient, and inexpensive way to solicit quotations. Usually, this method requires a call-back from the vendor, thus resulting in some time delays. Also, some type of written note should be maintained for future reference. Exhibit 4-2 is an example of a sample form that can be used for this procedure. This form is also useful for recording quotes received during vendor representative visits. Both telephone quotes and representative visits are appropriate for short-term or immediate needs and low-volume items.

Care must be exercised when soliciting telephone quotations to avoid mistakes and misunderstandings in regard to quantity required, manufacturer's product number, availability, pricing errors, and delivery requirements. These errors can be avoided by maintaining clear, concise information regarding the proposed purchase. Misunderstandings can occur at both ends of the telephone conversation, so it is wise to verify all necessary information regarding the transaction.

Exhibit 4-1 Sample Policy

```
                                                          POLICY
                                                          MMPD-002
                                                          7/3/79


                         ST. FRANCIS HOSPITAL
                         BLUE ISLAND,ILLINOIS

                         MATERIEL MANAGEMENT DEPARTMENT
                         PURCHASING DIVISION
                         COMPETITIVE BIDDING


                              POLICY
    The Purchasing Division shall seek competitive bids whenever feasible.


                             PROCEDURE
    I.  Competitive bids will be sought based upon the following criteria:

        A.  For supply items with an annual expenditure of $500.00 or more.
            and not covered under a group purchasing contract, yearly
            formal bids will be requested and submitted in writing.

        B.  For equipment with a unit cost of $150.00 to $300.00, bids
            will be requested by telephone to be submitted in writing.

        C.  For equipment with a unit cost of $300.00 or more, bids will be
            requested and submitted in writing.

        D.  For other purchases not categorized above, as deemed appropriate
            by the Director, Materiel Management or Purchasing Agent.

   II.  Formal bids will be requested from a minimum of three (3) vendors.
        Exceptions to this requirement must be approved by the Director,
        Materiel Management.

  III.  Vendors will be required to submit two copies of each bid requested.
        One copy to be filed with the Purchasing copy of the purchase order.
        The second copy to be filed in the closed bid file.

   IV.  Vendors will normally be given three (3) weeks to respond to written
        bids.

        A.  Vendors will be required to indicate the bid number on the outside
            of the mailing envelope.
        B.  Bids will be opened and evaluated on the morning of the next
            working day following the closing date.
        C.  Bids received after the closing date will not be considered without
            the approval of the Director.  Normal closing time for all bids
            will be 4:00 P.M. on the date specified.
```

Exhibit 4-1 continued

POLICY
MMPD-002
7/3/79
Page 2

V.   Bids for commodity classes or high volume items requiring drop shipments, may be awarded utilizing a blanket purchase order. These items are subject to the Purchasing Division procedure concerning blanket purchase orders.

VI. Bids awarded for items routinely ordered by departmental traveling requisitions shall be noted on each traveling requisition with the bid number and expiration date.

VII. Whenever practical, bids will be awarded for a period of at least one year.

_____

Director, Materiel Management

Exhibit 4-2 Working Bid Sheet

ST FRANCIS HOSPITAL	QUANTITY	UNIT	VENDORS				
DESCRIPTION							
DISCOUNT							
TERMS							
FOB							
DELIVERY							
NET PRICE							

For larger dollar volume supplies and equipment, a formal written quotation is more appropriate. Greater emphasis is being placed on cost documentation by third party payers and government programs, such as Medicare and Medicaid. Written documentation to substantiate costs is an absolute necessity. The burden of proof that a hospital uses competitive bidding and is obtaining the lowest cost possible rests with the purchasing department. Inquiries made by the third party intermediaries and administration no longer can be given lip service. Proper documentation is now, and probably forever will be, the name of the game for purchasing.

Because of these necessary documentation requirements, it is also advisable to maintain complete documentation for large-volume supplies or equipment that are purchased on the basis of sole source requirements or specific direction by the using department. When directed or sole source purchase requisitions are received, the practitioner should request a letter of justification from the user as well as administrative approval for these requests prior to the actual purchase. For nonrepetitive purchases, this documentation should be maintained with purchasing's copy of the purchase order. For repetitive purchases, a copy of the justification should be placed in the appropriate vendor file and renewed annually.

Basic Process

The first step in the bidding process is the evaluation of need (Chapter 2). Once the forecasted volume has been determined, the next step is to determine which vendors will be included in the bidding process. Naturally, you will want to include those vendors with a proven track record. However, consideration should also be given to every vendor possible, to eliminate potential claims of favoritism and provide for a broad range of responses. The third step is sending out the quotation forms. Depending upon what is included in the quotation, the participating vendors should be given two to three weeks to finalize and return their proposals.

Competitive bidding forms will vary with each hospital and specific situation. For situations involving standard items, a "request for quotation form" similar to Exhibit 4-3 can be used. These forms are relatively inexpensive, can be purchased locally, and can be personalized with the hospital name and address. This type of form has four parts with special carbons so that the vendor's name and address appear on only one of the copies (Exhibit 4-4). Specific spaces are provided for all necessary information. If the hospital has an extensive boilerplate (Chapter 1), the hospital's terms and conditions should be printed on the back of each of the bidder's copies. The addition of the boilerplate often will necessitate a custom printing that will substantially increase the form's cost; nevertheless, it should be included. From a legal standpoint, the quotation form is used to solicit a response to an offer. The hospital's terms and conditions are a substantial part of the transaction. They should be communicated to the vendor, who thus has the

Exhibit 4-3 Request for Quotation Form

ST. FRANCIS HOSPITAL
12935 SO. GREGORY STREET
BLUE ISLAND, ILLINOIS 60406

Request for
Quotation

NUMBER-

The above number must appear on all quotations and related correspondence.
THIS IS NOT AN ORDER

DATE	QUOTE NOT LATER THAN	REQUISITION NO.	DATE OF REQUISITION	CHARGEABLE ACCOUNT NUMBER(S)	P. O. NUMBER

VENDOR	ITEM	SUMMARY OF QUOTATIONS BY QUANTITY

DELIVERY REQUIREMENTS	DELIVERY PROMISED	TERMS	F.O.B.

ITEM	QUANTITY	DESCRIPTION	UNIT PRICE	AMOUNT

Buyer

REASON ORDER PLACED WITH SUCCESSFUL VENDOR	OTHER REASONS

Lowest Price   Quality   Best Del'y   Service   Only Source   Best Design

☐ ☐ ☐ ☐ ☐ ☐

Exhibit 4-4 Request for Quotation Form, Page 2

ST. FRANCIS HOSPITAL
12935 SO. GREGORY STREET
BLUE ISLAND, ILLINOIS 60406

Request for
Quotation

NUMBER-

The above number must appear on all quotations and related correspondence.
THIS IS NOT AN ORDER

DATE	QUOTE NOT LATER THAN	REQUISITION NO.	DATE OF REQUISITION	CHARGEABLE ACCOUNT NUMBER(S)	P. O. NUMBER

PLEASE QUOTE ON THIS SHEET IN SPACES INDICATED BELOW FOR THE ARTICLES DESCRIBED.
NOTE DELIVERY REQUIRED AND IN QUOTING, ADVISE DEFINITE DELIVERY.

BASE YOUR QUOTATIONS ON THE TERMS AND CONDITIONS PRINTED AND/OR TYPED HEREON.

WE QUOTE YOU AS BELOW

NAME OF COMPANY

BY (SIGNATURE)

OFFICIAL TITLE   QUOTATION DATE

DELIVERY REQUIREMENTS	DELIVERY PROMISED	TERMS	F.O.B.

ITEM	QUANTITY	DESCRIPTION	UNIT PRICE	AMOUNT

Buyer ——————————————

opportunity to accept or reject them. Further, inclusion of the terms and conditions can minimize problems during future negotiations.

For more complex quotations, the use of a letter may be more appropriate to present clear and concise information to the prospective vendors. Specific projects may entail the necessity for extensive and detailed specifications. Appendix 4-A is provided as an illustration. As you will note, the sample specifications are for a microfilming proposal. As a general rule, the more complex the project, the more detailed the specification should be.

Within the competitive bidding process, open or closed procedures can be utilized. The open procedure means that vendors are permitted to be present when the bids are opened. The open bid process is most often utilized when there is no doubt that the lowest bidder will receive the order. If quality, quantity, and vendor analyses have been completed, price is the only remaining factor to be determined. Therefore, awarding to the low bidder should not cause any problem.

When the closed procedure is used, vendors are not permitted at the bid opening, but are informed of the results after a decision has been finalized. Of the two procedures, the closed procedure is the more popular among hospital purchasing practitioners.

Regardless of which procedure is employed, care should be taken when analyzing the proposals. A common mistake made in the evaluation process is to concentrate on unit cost and ignore payment discounts and freight charges. The following illustration will help to clarify this point.

	Vendor A	Vendor B
Discount on list price	23%	21%
Payment terms	Net 30	2½% ten days; net 30 days
FOB point	Hospital	Shipping point

To the inexperienced practitioner, vendor B appears to be the low bidder based upon a total discount of 23½ percent (21 percent plus 2½ percent prompt payment terms). However, the difference in FOB point could be the deciding factor. Vendor A indicates FOB hospital, whereas vendor B indicates FOB shipping point. Vendor B's quotation means the hospital will pay all freight costs. Depending upon the actual shipping point, the freight charges could offset or be higher than the difference between the discounts offered. Before the actual award can be made, it will be necessary to determine actual freight costs to arrive at the actual net cost. Only when the total net cost for both vendors is known can the low bid be determined and an award made.

DISCOUNTS

In the health care marketplace usually two types of discounts are available—quantity and cash. Quantity discounts are of two types: (1) specific quantities in connection with a single purchase; and (2) discounts involving quantities estimated to cover the hospital's requirements for a specific period of time. Quantity discounts on a particular purchase refer to the fact that the larger the quantity ordered, the lower the price per unit. In evaluating this type of discount, one must consider the possible impact of a large quantity on inventory costs. An increased quantity discount will lower the unit cost, but it may increase holding costs, thus resulting in an uneconomical purchase over the long term.

Quantity discounts covering a specified period of time are advantageous for both the hospital and the vendor. The vendor is sure of the hospital's business for a specific period of time (usually six months to one year) and for an estimated quantity. The hospital has some assurance of a reliable source of supply at a good price for the same specified time period.

Cash discounts, or prompt payment terms, result in a lower net cost to the hospital. The accounting department is responsible for meeting payment terms, but purchasing practitioners should be sure to include the terms on the purchase order and to advise accounting. This can be simply accomplished by using a rubber stamp stating "Discount Terms" on accounting's copy of the purchase order. Purchasing practitioners should also clearly define when the discount period begins. The notation of "2 percent ten days; net 30" is less than adequate. A more appropriate statement would be "a 2 percent discount will be taken for invoice payment within ten days of receipt of merchandise." As a general rule, purchasing practitioners should include this type of statement on the hospital quotation form and allow the vendor to modify it if desired. The axiom of "it never hurts to ask" applies here.

NEGOTIATION

Negotiation can be defined as proposing terms of accommodation with respect to the purchase or sale of goods or services. Negotiation is not haggling over the price, as is common in many open air markets. Nor is it an attempt by the buyer to play one vendor against another to drive prices down. Negotiation is a process, an art and technique, of arriving at a common understanding through bargaining on the essentials of a purchase, such as specifications, delivery, price, and terms.

Every purchasing practitioner needs good negotiation skills and should begin to learn proper techniques early. The lack of sound negotiation skill by practitioners is the primary reason why many department heads act as quasi-purchasing agents, since they feel as skilled as the purchasing agent who has little, if any, formal training in this critical discipline.

The negotiation process should be used selectively because it is often lengthy and very costly. Typical areas in which the process can be effectively applied are:

- price as it relates to the terms and conditions of a competitive bid or proposal

- changes in delivery points (FOB), method of delivery (UPS or common carrier), or packaging

- variations in quality or price originally agreed upon

- escalator clauses

- when supplies or services are available only from one vendor

- ˙contracts of extended duration

- when no acceptable bids have been received from responsible vendors

- when it is impractical to draft exact specifications or detailed descriptions of certain supplies or services

- when termination of a previously agreed-to contract is desired or considered necessary by the hospital

Basic Process

Preparation

The negotiation process begins with the preparation or prenegotiation planning stage. Before negotiations can begin, it is important to set specific goals of what is to be achieved.

Within the goal-setting process specific needs should be expressed, such as terms and conditions, delivery time, and FOB. Without defining needs in specific terms, your ability to prepare for and conduct negotiations will be seriously impaired. Once the needs are defined, you should establish a level of expectation you hope to achieve during the actual negotiations. Negotiators who set high levels of expectation (lower prices, better delivery) tend to be more successful than negotiators with lower levels of expectation. Aim high, and once you set your level of expectation, stay with it.

After defining the specific needs and expectations, you can begin to define clearly the specific goals to be achieved. In setting goals, two important criteria should be remembered. Goals must be realistic, and they must be supportable. Even goals set with a high expectation level can be supported; perhaps they are not as supportable as lower goals, but they are supportable nevertheless.

Once goals have been established, they may have to be reviewed and approved by administration and, perhaps, by the board. This is often the case for purchasing practitioners because of dollar limitations or levels of commitment imposed by administration. Typical examples include a $500 unit cost or only items specifically expressed in the operating or capital budgets. Armed with the necessary authority to proceed, the goals become the foundation around which ranges of settlement can be determined.

The range of settlement refers to the maximum and minimum positions that are acceptable to you. As a purchasing practitioner, the minimum position represents your initial position upon entering the negotiations. For example, if upon entering a negotiation session for interior decorating services you were to state something to the effect that "the proposal had absolutely no value to you or the hospital," you would clearly state your minimum position. Any concessions should be made upward toward your highest level of expectation or your maximum position. It is important that both the maximum and minimum positions be supportable by fact and logic.

Analysis of Supplier Position

Now that you have an established position, it is important to understand the vendor's position. Normally, the vendor's stated goals are contained in the proposal. Through a careful comparison of your goals and the vendor's proposal, you should be able to discern areas of disagreement. As part of your review, the vendor's proposal should also be subjected to value analysis, that is, the price proposed in relation to the value of the item or service to be purchased. A complete cost analysis should also be conducted to determine what, if any, latitude the vendor may have in cost reduction. Value analysis and cost analysis can be most beneficial to your position and supportive of your expectations. For example, if you are dealing with a custom-made surgical pack for open heart surgery, it would be wise to ask the vendor to provide a complete cost analysis of how the unit cost was arrived at. Vendors may not be willing (sometimes not even able) to provide you with this information, but it never hurts to ask.

Terms and conditions of the vendor proposal should be closely examined. In almost every instance, all terms and conditions are subject to negotiation despite claims to the contrary from the vendor representative. For example, many vendors prefer to submit proposals on their standard sales forms. Close examination of the terms and conditions printed on the reverse side will reveal that they protect the vendor and effectively negate the terms and conditions on the hospital's purchase order.

During negotiations with a *Fortune 500* company for some major capital equipment, the negotiating team of a small 105-bed community hospital successfully negotiated terms and conditions that were mutually beneficial to both sides. The company maintained many of its original terms and conditions and the hospital had terms and conditions added to the standard sales contract that provided the protection that the hospital sought. Not only was the hospital successful, but as a result of this experience, the company (which had the health care industry targeted as a new market) revised its terms and conditions on its standard sales agreement in an effort to reduce future negotiating costs and to improve the company's marketing strategy. Realistically, these results are not an everyday occurrence but they do prove two things: (1) vendors' terms and conditions can be negotiated; and (2) high levels of expectations can be attained if you are persistent.

When dealing with contracts for items with alternative substitutes, every effort should be made to become familiar with those items and their associated costs. This can be accomplished by reading technical literature, by visiting other hospitals, and through discussions with technical experts on the hospital staff. The greater your knowledge, the more you can increase support for your position.

It is further advisable to learn as much as possible about the vendor's negotiator(s). During the bidding process, your dealings are normally with the representative. However, during a negotiation you can expect the representative to appear with the general manager, or even a vice-president. Make sure your opponent has the necessary authority to negotiate and commit to the contract.

The final step in the preparation stage is to prepare a strategy. At this time there are three major tasks to be completed. The first is to develop arguments and counterarguments by using the data collected. Not only should you support your position, but you should try to anticipate the vendor's defense against your position and in support of the vendor's. A useful technique for preparation is to have other members of the purchasing department or the requesting department head rehearse with you. The use of a devil's advocate is often helpful here.

The second task is to try to anticipate the vendor's range of settlement. Remember, the original proposal contains the vendor's high expectation. The vendor's low or minimum position has not been stated. One easy technique is to talk to other hospitals or local businesses that the vendor serves to find out what they are paying for similar products or services.

The final task is to prepare an agenda listing the topics to be discussed. The agenda should be arranged with your most powerful arguments presented first, your weakest arguments next, and your best arguments last. Psychologists refer to this as the primacy-recency effect. The primacy effect relates the fact that some people tend to retain information presented early in the discussion. The recency effect states that whatever is said last will be remembered best. Logically, you want to place your weakest arguments in the middle because they are most often forgotten first. Just remember, the vendor is also aware of the primacy-recency effect and will use it on you.

Techniques

Negotiation techniques will vary depending upon the situation and your level of expectation. Early in the negotiation session every effort should be made to express mutual interest. Reinforcement of this position may be necessary from time to time to remind the vendor that the objective of the discussion is to obtain an agreement in the best interests of both the vendor and the hospital. Conveying the feeling that the hospital welcomes the vendor as a member of the team provides a sense of participation and "wanting to help."

Listening can be one of the most important techniques a skilled negotiator can use. Often the vendor will feel the need to respond to your silence by talking. The more you can get the vendor to talk, the greater the possibility of gaining information relative to the vendor's range of settlement and overall position.

Asking questions will aid in obtaining information. The use of questions is also valuable to divert attention from an area you are not fully prepared to discuss, to place the vendor on the defensive, to elicit support for the vendor's position, and, finally, to help the vendor to accept your position.

The preparation of alternative positions is another technique that can provide a measure of success. The use of this technique can serve three purposes:

1. Obtaining information by sending up a trial balloon. By offering an extreme position, you may be able to learn the vendor's actual level of expectation.
2. Problem solving. By offering an alternative solution, you may find an area of compromise. Remember, you should only offer those alternatives that are totally acceptable to you.
3. Breaking an impasse. It is not uncommon for some type of impasse to occur during negotiation and it should be anticipated.

Humor has a valid place in negotiation. It can best be utilized to divert direct confrontation and relax tensions. As a negotiation technique, humor can also be used to withdraw or divert the vendor when the vendor is concentrating on an argument that you may not be prepared to deal with—except, perhaps, when some concession is involved, which brings us to the next technique.

Making concessions during negotiations requires careful consideration and timing. As a technique, concession should be used (1) to break an impasse, (2) to win a corresponding concession from the vendor, and (3) to conclude an agreement.

Making a concession should be treated as making a trade. Always trade upward; concede on a minor point to win a major point. As a general rule, concessions should not be made early in the session, lest you give the impression that you are an "easy" negotiator. This technique is best saved for the middle or end of the session to show your sincerity regarding mutual interest.

In team negotiation situations, the use of role playing, known as "good guy/bad guy," may be an effective technique. This technique requires that the "bad guy" assume an extreme position that might impose a serious threat to the vendor. The "good guy" assumes a more reasonable position, one that the team is actually striving for. By disagreeing with the "bad guy" and, perhaps, even supporting the vendor, the "good guy" should attempt to win the confidence of the vendor and increase the chances of attaining the team's objective.

When this technique is utilized against you, ignore the "bad guy" and concentrate on effectively responding to the "good guy's" position and arguments. If the "bad guy" becomes too disruptive to the session, suggest that the "bad guy" leave or negotiations will have to be suspended temporarily.

The last technique is the use of a deadline date by which an agreement must be reached. This is probably the one technique that vendors utilize effectively. "If you order today you can save 10 percent because there will be a price increase effective tomorrow" is a typical example. What the vendor is trying to do is arrive at a quick agreement, and one that is probably unfavorable for you. In 99 of 100 cases, the deadline date is more imaginary than real. When a vendor really wants your business, whether the deadline date is real or not, the vendor can often hold the price for "a couple of days." When negotiating from the hospital position, deadline dates should be used only when they are real. It is often unwise to try a deadline date as a bluff. Unless you are a skilled negotiator, you may paint yourself into the proverbial corner and end up making concessions you had not planned.

As a final point on technique, the use of threats should have no place in purchasing negotiations. Threats are risky and can incur a high cost in the long run. As a practical matter, threats should be replaced by good solid data and logic to support your position.

Individual versus Team

Typically, hospital purchasing practitioners function as individual negotiators. However, there are occasions when the team concept may be practical and worthwhile. The purchase of laundry services is a good example. The executive housekeeper usually has greater knowledge of the technological processes involved than the purchasing practitioner does. When a situation such as this arises, the team concept comes into play. A team leader must then be chosen. And since the leader should be the team member with the best negotiation skills, this should always be the purchasing practitioner. The team leader plays a vital role in the negotiations, not only as a spokesperson for the team, but also as mediator, unifier, and consolidator. The team leader must take the various individual opinions of the team and create a solid, unified position.

Moreover, each team member must recognize and support the leader's role as spokesperson for the group. For this reason, team members should also be chosen with care, on the basis of what each can specifically contribute to the actual negotiations.

When utilizing the team concept, it is particularly important that all team members be involved in the preparation process from the outset. Each team member should be totally familiar with goals and strategy. One of the most disastrous effects of a poorly prepared team can be the lack of proper presentation of information or position to the vendor's representatives.

Each team member should be responsible for specific areas or sections to be negotiated. For instance, if negotiating for laundry services, the housekeeper may be responsible for washing and processing requirements, while the purchasing practitioner may handle pricing and delivery schedules. By having designated areas of responsibility, the team members present the psychological impression to the vendor of a solid, unified front representing all areas affected by the contract.

A technique that is often employed in team negotiations is the caucus. A caucus can be used to:

- evaluate new information presented by the vendor

- evaluate concessions by the vendor

- restore calm if an emotional situation presents itself

- divert attention away from an area that one is unprepared for or that may require a concession

- gain additional information in support of an important point

The caucus is a useful technique and should be employed as necessary. No matter how careful and complete your preparation, something new will probably be presented during the actual negotiations that was not anticipated.

Concluding the Agreement

When a satisfactory agreement appears imminent, a suggestion to wrap up should be made. When the vendor makes this recommendation, be sure you are prepared to accept the agreement. The final agreement should be reviewed to be sure that all agreements reached during the negotiations are understood by both parties. Often an area or issue on which one of the parties thought agreement had been reached, but it actually had not, may surface. Whenever this happens, the problem must be resolved immediately.

Sometimes it is beneficial to have purchase orders pretyped, setting forth possible agreements that are expected to be concluded. In any event, the purchasing secretary should be prepared to type the final agreement. Once completed, the final agreement should be reviewed and signed by both parties. If the agreement is to be prepared by the vendor, it should be reviewed carefully to ensure that the contract reflects the understandings agreed upon. If an agreement cannot be signed immediately, a memorandum of understanding should be prepared that shows the exact wording of any agreements reached, and it should be signed by both parties.

When the final contract is presented, it should be carefully compared with the memorandum of understanding. If the contract is in order, sign it and conclude the negotiations.

EFFECTIVE UTILIZATION OF GROUP PURCHASING

Group purchasing is a concept that is based upon the principle that together the member hospitals have greater purchasing power than would any individual member acting alone. Through group purchasing it should be possible for the group collectively to negotiate lower prices from the vendor. And this very often is the case, especially in large metropolitan areas. Religious groups, such as the Sisters of Mercy in Chicago and Detroit, the Sisters of St. Mary in St. Louis, and the Consortium of Jewish Hospitals (a nationwide group based in Chicago), have also achieved a large measure of success in their group purchasing efforts.

However, the group purchasing concept does have some pitfalls of which practitioners should be aware. First, group purchasing assumes that all its members agree to use brand X. If your institution prefers brand Y, you cannot take advantage of the group contract.

Second, suppliers who did not win a group contract sometimes will reduce their prices to induce individual members not to utilize the contract.

And third, larger hospitals sometimes strike out on their own and competitively bid their larger volume items to achieve a lower price.

Such pitfalls tend to have only one result; they weaken the collective bargaining position of the group. Every practitioner is faced with any or all of these pitfalls at one time or another, and must deal with them. As a practitioner, this author has had the opportunity to work in both large and small hospitals. There is little doubt that the large hospital provides the necessary volume to help the small hospital achieve the benefits of group purchasing. While working in the small hospital, this author appreciated the efforts of the large hospital in its support of the group. While working at the large hospital, the author did not forget the influence the large hospital has on the group effort. As a general practice, group purchasing contracts have always had first priority. When brand X is not acceptable, every effort must be made to determine why this is so. Once the basis for brand X's unacceptability has been determined, this information should be transmitted to the group office with a recommendation to explore the possibility of changing manufacturers.

When dealing with a vendor who is undercutting the group contract, you should inform the representative that every consideration has been given to the new offer, and that you would like the other members of the group to share in the offer and so you are forwarding a copy to the group office for further negotiations. If that does not shock your vendor into reality concerning the strength of the group, then it is doubtful that anything will.

If you are the practitioner at a large hospital (300 or more beds) remember that by withdrawing your volume from the group contract you will only hurt the ability of the group to gain negotiating strength at contract renewal. While the large hospital may not be adversely affected by a significant price increase, the small hospitals in the group will be. Undercutting the group contract leads to higher prices for everyone.

Finally, as a member of a group, you should encourage firm commitment of volume contracts. Marketing representatives tend to make concessions when they know what the anticipated volume of the group is for a given period and that they can be assured of not losing that volume. Many groups have found this to be a highly successful tactic in negotiating group contracts.

In the last analysis, group purchasing is only as successful as the individual purchasing practitioner makes it. Group purchasing is a sound procedure to use and should be supported.

APPENDIX 4-A

Sample Specification

November 9, 1979

RE: Invitation to bid—MICROFILM SERVICES BID # 106

Gentlemen:

St. Francis Hospital invites you to submit a quotation for microfilm services as described in hospital's specification herein attached.

Bidder's proposal shall be submitted on a net cost per thousand images. Net cost shall include all labor costs for preparation of material; film and/or fiche costs; fiche indexing costs; packing cartons; transportation; and document destruction. If, at bidder's option, a proposal is submitted on a basis other than net cost per thousand, each component of cost (as listed above) must include bidder's estimate of each component and must be extended to arrive at an estimated total cost.

Bidder's proposal shall be submitted indicating type of record, cost per thousand, and total cost. This should follow the detail given in sections II-VI of hospital's specification.

The term of this proposal shall be for a period of one year from date of hospital's purchase order. Hospital desires price protection for the term of the contract.

Bidder's proposal shall include all applicable cash terms and anticipated delivery time for microforms from date of pickup of hospital's records.

Bidder's proposal shall include identification of the type and manufacturer of the equipment to be utilized in the filming procedure. The manufacturer of the roll film and fiche to be used shall also be included.

Bidder's proposal shall include at least three references of hospitals who have or are currently utilizing bidder's services.

References shall include hospital name, complete address, telephone number and person to be contacted.

Bidders may review all records, if desired, by contacting the undersigned for an appointment at 312-597-2000 extension 5311.

St. Francis Hospital is a not-for-profit institution exempt from the Retailers' Occupation Tax, the Service Occupation Tax and the Service Use Tax.

Bidder shall submit his proposal in duplicate. Proposals shall be submitted in a sealed envelope indicating the bid number on the face of the envelope.

Proposals will be due in the office of Edward D. Sanderson, Director, Materiel Management, St. Francis Hospital, 12935 S. Gregory Street, Blue Island, Illinois, 60406 by 4:00 P.M. on Wednesday, December 12, 1979.

Bids will be opened on Thursday, December 13, 1979, with an evaluation and review process to follow.

Hospital reserves the right to reject any and all bids or any part thereof.

Very truly yours,

For St. Francis Hospital

Edward D. Sanderson
Director, Materiel Management

EDS/mq
Enclosure

ST. FRANCIS HOSPITAL
MICROFILM BID SPECIFICATION

SCOPE OF THE PROJECT: This project encompasses filming and/or fiche for various records in the Business Office, Accounting, Payroll, Personnel and Medical Records Departments of St. Francis Hospital. Each of these departments is detailed separately within this document. General instructions contained herein apply to all filming to be completed as part of this project.

SECTION I   GENERAL

A. *PREPARATION PROCEDURE*

Preparation of records, as described below, will be performed by the contractor. Preparation procedure will consist of:

1. The entire file will be reviewed in order to verify the correctness of the filing arrangement. All misfiled cases will be filed in their proper sequence.

2. All wire staples, paper clips and other impediments which might hinder the microfilming operation will be removed from the records. Worn or torn documents will be repaired to ensure the complete legibility of the resultant microfilms.

B. *MICROFILM PROCEDURE—ROLL FILM*

1. The film used will be high resolution permanent type microfilm. The processed microfilm will contain a triangle in the margin indicating that the film meets Federal Standards for permanence, as specified in American National Standards PH 1.28.

2. All processed microfilm will contain less than 0.005 milligram per square inch of residual ammonium or sodium thiosulfate (hypo), and will meet American National Standards PH 4.8 for archival permanence.

3. Each film roll shall contain not less than 18 inches of film leader and 18 inches of film trailer. It is understood that the hospital will, at its option, take film rolls at random and submit short strips of film, taken from the leader or trailer, to an independent laboratory for testing as per (a) above.

4. The background density of the processed microfilm images shall be not less than 0.9 or more than 1.3 diffuse transmission density. This measurement will be made in accordance with American National Standards PH 2.17 and PH 2.19.

5. The resolution of the completed microfilm shall be not less than 80 lines per millimeter as determined by using National Bureau of Standards Microcopy Test Chart No. 1010a. Resolution is the result of high quality cameras, lens, and film. The camera must be in proper adjustment and high quality processing is also required.

6. The following identification and indexing targets will be used on each roll of microfilm.

    (a) *START* target—in large letters, identifiable with the naked eye.
    (b) Title target, including the name of the hospital, type of records and beginning case number, patient name, employee name, or company name as may be applicable.
    (c) *END* title target showing date records were filmed, camera operator's signature and description of roll contents, including number of film images appearing thereon as determined by automatic machine count of documents filmed.

7. After completion of the microfilming operation, exposed film will be developed, after which each film roll will be given at least two inspections to ensure complete legibility of every image appearing thereon. In the event that any document within a chart is not legible, all of the documents comprising the chart will be rephotographed and spliced to the end of the film roll. Any retakes that may be required will be at the expense of the contractor.

8. Each film roll will be housed in a cardboard container to which will be affixed an indexing label. This label will include the roll number, complete index of contents, and the name of the hospital.

C. *MICROFILM PROCEDURE (UNITIZED)—FICHE*

1. Depending upon the type of fiche process offered, the requirements noted in Section B, paragraphs 1, 2, 4, 5, and 7 will apply.
2. The contractor shall furnish fiche, size 4 × 6 inches.

D. *DOCUMENT PICK-UP*

The contractor will supply packing cartons for the records at no extra charge All records shall be packed for shipment by contractor's personnel.

E. *DELIVERY*

The contractor agrees to have all work completed and microfilms delivered to the hospital within approximately 45 working days after records are taken into his custody.

F. *DESTRUCTION OF ORIGINAL RECORDS*

Unless otherwise instructed by the hospital, the contractor will arrange to destroy all original documents after the hospital has approved the film. The documents must be destroyed by shredding or burning. The contractor will furnish the hospital with a notarized certification attesting to the destruction of the original records.

Hospital agrees to complete a thorough inspection of the film within two weeks after receipt.

G. *REFERENCE*

If the hospital has need for emergency reference to any record that is in the custody of the contractor, the hospital is entitled to telephone "collect" privileges to contact the contractor's laboratory as many times as required. The contractor shall provide such reference service 24 hours a day, 7 days a week. The records shall be maintained in an accessible fashion so that emergency telephone reference may be obtained within one hour, during normal business hours, and within two hours at any other time.

H. *BILLING PROCEDURE*

The contractor may invoice the hospital as completed microfilm is delivered to the hospital. All invoices rendered shall be accompanied by a detailed work sheet showing the following information about each film roll:

1. reel number
2. contents (beginning to ending record numbers; patient or employee names; dates of computer runs; and/or firm names as applicable)
3. number of images on the film roll

It is understood that the hospital will, during its inspection of completed work, select at random one or more rolls, count the images produced, and verify the accuracy of the total count.

All invoices will be submitted in duplicate, marked to the attention of Director, Materiel Management.

I. *GUARANTEE*

The contractor guarantees that the microforms will be produced in a manner as prescribed herein. The hospital reserves the right to reject any portion or all of the microforms produced by the contractor that do not meet the specifications and terms of this proposal. The hospital, at its option, may then demand that the work be done over according to specifications, or may elect to reject the work, retaining all microforms produced which do not meet specifications and withhold payment for same.

SECTION II　MEDICAL RECORDS DEPARTMENT

A. *MEDICAL RECORDS FOR YEARS 1958-1968*

There are approximately 95,500 records, averaging 51 images each, comprising an estimated total of 4,870,500 images. These charts are filed in serial unit sequence. These charts have been purged and except for staple removal are ready for filming.

These records are to be in a roll film format. The front portion of each chart is to be filmed. A divider target, to be agreed upon at the time of contract award, is to be placed between each unit record. Both the front of the chart and divider target are included in the above images/record and total images.

B. *MEDICAL RECORDS—PATIENT DECEASED*

There are approximately 5,100 records, averaging 195 images each, comprising an estimated total of 994,500 total images. These records are maintained in terminal digit sequence, and have not been purged.

These records are to be in a roll film format. The front portion of each chart is to be filmed. A divider target, to be agreed upon at the time of contract award, is to be placed between each unit record. Both the front of the chart and divider target are included in the above images/record and total images.

C. MEDICAL RECORDS FOR YEARS 1969-1972

There are approximately 15,200 records, averaging 195 images each, comprising an estimated total of 2,964,000 total images. These records are maintained in terminal digit sequence and have not been purged.

These records are to be in a microfiche format. Each "unit" fiche will be identified at the top with the unit number, last name, first name, and middle initial of the patient. The word "Admission" and a date (i.e., 01-01-69) will be used as targets to indicate a break in the unit record. The front of the chart will be filmed and placed as the first image. Both the front of the chart and the divider target have been included in the above images/record and total images.

SECTION III   PATIENT ACCOUNTS

A. INPATIENT RECORDS

There are approximately 50,000 charts, averaging 30 images each, comprising an estimated total of 1,500,000 images encompassing the years of 1976, 1977, and 1978. These records are maintained in alphabetical sequence by year.

These records are to be in a roll film format. The front portion of each chart envelope is to be filmed. A divider target, to be agreed upon at the time of contract award, is to be placed between each individual record. Both the envelope front and divider target are included in the above images/record and total images.

B. OUTPATIENT RECORDS

There are approximately 160,000 charts, averaging 9 images each, comprising an estimated total of 1,440,000 images encompassing the years 1976, 1977, and 1978. These records are maintained in alphabetical sequence by year.

These records are to be in a roll film format. The front portion of each chart envelope is to be filmed. A divider target, to be agreed upon at the time of contract award, is to be placed between each individual record. Both the envelope front and divider target are included in the above images/record and total images.

C. CASH RECEIPT POSTING TICKETS

There are approximately 200 tickets/day $\times$ 365 days $\times$ 7 years equalling an estimated total of 511,000 images encompassing the years 1971-1978. These tickets are maintained by day.

These tickets are to be in a roll film format. A divider target indicating month, day, and year (e.g., 01-01-71) is to be placed at the start of each day's tickets. The divider target is included in the above total images.

D. *INCOME DAILY SUMMARY REPORTS*

These are computer generated reports averaging 300 pages per day × 365 days × 3 years equaling an estimated total of 328,500 images encompassing the years 1976, 1977, and 1978. This report is maintained by day.

These reports are to be in a roll film format. A divider target indicating month, day, and year (e.g., 01-01-76) is to be placed at the start of each day's listings. The divider target is included in the above total images.

SECTION IV   PERSONNEL DEPARTMENT

A. There are approximately 1,800 personnel records, averaging 10 images each, comprising an estimated total of 18,000 images encompassing the years 1973-1977. These records have been stripped and are to be totally filmed including the face of the file folder. These records are maintained in alphabetical sequence by year.

These records are to be in a roll film format. A divider target indicating the letter of the alphabet is to be used and should be large enough to be clearly understood.

The contractor will provide a typewritten listing of all records contained on a specific roll of film. This listing will include last name, first name, middle initial, and employee number as indicated on the label used for identification of the record folder.

B. *MISCELLANEOUS COMPUTER REPORTS*

There are five separate reports on computer paper comprising an estimated total of 2,651 images encompassing the years 1974-1978. These reports are yearly summaries.

These records are to be in microfiche format. Fiche identification will be determined at the time of contract award.

The following reports are to be on fiche:

Budget Variance
1974-76 pages   1977-79 pages
1975-79 pages   1978-83 pages
1976-80 pages

Payroll Master Proof
1975-127 pages   1977-209 pages
1976-129 pages   1978-214 pages

Personnel Budgets
1974-109 pages   1977-195 pages
1975-171 pages   1978-199 pages
1976-192 pages

Pension Year-to-Date Contributions
1977- 33 pages
1978- 22 pages
1979-573 pages

Salary Scales
1971- 3 pages   1976-12 pages
1972- 3 pages   1977-16 pages
1973- 3 pages   1978-13 pages
1974- 3 pages   1979-14 pages
1975-14 pages

SECTION V   PAYROLL DEPARTMENT

A. There are approximately 70,200 time cards, at two images each (front and back), comprising an estimated total of 140,400 images encompassing the years 1974-1978. These records are maintained in alphabetical sequence by department number, by pay period by year.

These records are to be in a roll film format. A divider target indicating month, day, and year (e.g., 01-01-76) is to be placed at the start of each pay period's time cards. There are 26 pay periods per year.

B. *MISCELLANEOUS COMPUTER REPORTS*

There are five separate reports on computer paper, comprising an estimated total of 46,300 images encompassing the years 1974-1978. These reports are maintained by pay period.

These records are to be in a microfiche format. Fiche identification will include report name 'and date.

The following reports are to be on fiche:

YEARS 1974-1977

Year-to-Date Reports	-	35 pages/report	26/year
Payroll Register	-	80 pages/report	26/year
Deduction Register	-	40 pages/report	12/year
Master Proof Reports	-	215 pages/report	26/year

		1978	
Year-to-Date Reports	-	35 pages/report	26/year
Payroll Register	-	80 pages/report	26/year
Deduction Register	-	40 pages/report	26/year
Master Proof Reports	-	215 pages/report	26/year
Quarter-to-Date			
Reports	-	110 pages/report	4/year

SECTION VI   ACCOUNTING DEPARTMENT

A. *ACCOUNTS PAYABLE RECORDS*

There are approximately 40,000 vouchers, averaging 10 images each, comprising an estimated total of 400,000 images, encompassing the years 1974-1977. These records are maintained in consecutive number sequence by year.

These records are to be in a roll film format. There will *not* be a divider target between vouchers. Years are to be kept separately on film. There will only be one year or part of a year per roll.

Chapter 5

Ordering Systems

The daily, routine clerical demands of hospital purchasing often consume the time that should be devoted to planning and management. These clerical hours can be considerably out of proportion to the benefits derived. As much as 70 percent of a practitioner's time can be consumed by processing rush orders, repetitive small orders, and routine paperwork.

Experienced practitioners have recognized this problem and have developed time-saving systems to overcome or minimize it; a number of these are reviewed in the discussion that follows. Use of any of these systems should free time for the practitioner to devote to high dollar items and research. Without this time, there can be but limited opportunities for important cost containment activities.

STANDARD PURCHASE ORDER

The oldest ordering format used by practitioners is the straight fixed price purchase order. The standard purchase order states those terms and conditions the practitioner believes are necessary to describe the item(s) ordered and to establish a formal contract with the vendor. The format and specifics of the standard purchase order were covered in Chapter 1. The systems that follow are basically variations of the use of the standard purchase order.

TELEPHONE ORDERS

Placing orders via the telephone is quick, easy, and efficient. Pricing and delivery can be determined immediately by the practitioner. Telephone ordering also may eliminate the necessity for forwarding a confirmation copy of the purchase order, and thus save at least part of the postage costs. Sending confirmation copies for telephone orders also increases the possibility of duplicate shipments.

Telephone ordering does not eliminate the need for typing a purchase order for internal hospital use. The purchase order provides the necessary documentation required to process receiving and payment, and to confirm the order placed. Typically, errors can be made by either the practitioner or the vendor in regard to quantities ordered, product description, and unit pricing. Thus, the typed purchase order becomes the basis for potential problem solving.

Another of the problems associated with telephone orders is that they may not be covered by the hospital's terms and conditions. This problem can be lessened by sending the vendor a copy of the terms and conditions and noting that all telephone orders are subject to the terms contained therein. As a rule, it is wise to have the vendor acknowledge, in writing, receipt of and agreement to the terms and conditions. This procedure should be completed annually or when the hospital's terms and conditions are modified in any way.

BLANKET ORDERS

A blanket purchase order provides for the vendor to furnish the item(s) indicated for a specific period of time and at a prearranged price. (See Exhibit 5-1.) The blanket order is an efficient means of reducing the number of small routine orders. Most often, ordering becomes a matter of notifying the vendor by telephone as requirements arise. Applications include orders for radioisotopes, typewriter repairs, routine office supplies, and repair parts.

The use of blanket orders offers a number of advantages:

- Increased volume, by combining requirements for a number of items, usually leads to increased savings over individual purchases.

- Pricing is often protected by the vendor for the term of the agreement.

- Ordering items as required effectively reduces the need for hospital-based inventory.

- Assuring the vendor of projected requirements affords the vendor the opportunity for efficient planning and reduced operating costs, which can be passed on to the hospital in the form of lower pricing and faster, if not improved, delivery.

Blanket orders require a specialized control system and improved communication. The simplest system is the call register (see Exhibit 5-2). As requirements arise, call numbers are assigned to individual requisitions. As described in Chapter 1, the four-part direct purchase requisition can be utilized to fill the documentation requirements. Part 1 can be maintained with purchasing's copy of the blanket order. Part 2 can be sent to accounting with the proper notation of the call number used. And Part 3 can be sent to receiving and utilized as a receiving report.

Exhibit 5-1 Special Receiving Document for Blanket Orders

ST. FRANCIS HOSPITAL
BLUE ISLAND, ILLINOIS

RECEIVING DEPARTMENT
BLANKET PURCHASE ORDER RELEASES

VENDOR _____   DATE WRITTEN _____

P.O. NUMBER _____   DATE EXPIRES _____

CALL NR,	DATE	ITEM DESCRIPTION	QUANTITY	DEPARTMENT	

Exhibit 5-2 Blanket Purchase Order Call Register

ST. FRANCIS HOSPITAL
BLUE ISLAND, ILLINOIS

PURCHASONG DEPARTMENT
BLANKET PURCHASE ORDER RELEASES

VENDOR _____   DATE WRITTEN _____

P.O. NUMBER _____   DATE EXPIRES _____

                                              MAXIMUM AMOUNT _____

CALL NR.	DATE	ITEM DESCRIPTION	DEPARTMENT	TOTAL $ VALUE	DOLLARS REMAINING

STANDING ORDERS

This form of blanket order usually directs the vendor to deliver specific quantities of merchandise on a predetermined time schedule. Use of the standing order eliminates the need to call the vendor to release every shipment. However, one of its disadvantages is that fluctuations in usage tend to increase or decrease delivery requirements. Either situation usually places a burden on the vendor in terms of rush deliveries or out-of-stock or overstock situations. This is especially true for orders covering custom-made products. One way to reduce rush deliveries and out-of-stock situations is to request the vendor to maintain an agreed-upon safety stock at the vendor's facility. To prevent or reduce the likelihood of vendor overstocks, the vendor should be notified as soon as possible when an overstock situation becomes apparent at the hospital. In most cases, custom-made products are normally set up for production just prior to the agreed-upon delivery date. Thus, the sooner you can notify the vendor, prior to the normal delivery date, the better your relationship with the vendor will be.

Standing orders are normally issued on a standard purchase order, which is typed to reflect the total annual quantity anticipated to be purchased. The purchase order is distributed as described in Chapter 1. The procedures for receiving and accounts payable are slightly altered with the standing order. When the merchandise is received, the receiving department annotates the purchase order with the amount and date received. A copy is created for both purchasing and accounts payable, signifying receipt of the release. Accounts payable matches the vendor's invoice with the payables copy of the receiving report and processes for payment.

CONSIGNMENT ORDERS

Consignment normally involves the maintaining of an inventory of the vendor's merchandise in the hospital. Ownership title does not pass to the hospital until the merchandise is withdrawn from the consignment stock. Most vendors are hesitant to agree to consignment arrangements, principally because of their concern for proper accounting by the hospital. Improper accounting usually occurs because of unauthorized withdrawals from inventory at night, or on weekends, by nonstoreroom employees.

Practitioners who are considering consignment inventories should give careful thought to the following points. First, the vendor must clearly identify all merchandise for consignment inventory. Second, the consignment inventory may need to be segregated from the regular inventory, if such an inventory exists. Third, the vendor and the hospital need to clarify insurance responsibility in case of fire and theft. And it is very difficult to identify theft as such because of unauthorized withdrawals. Fourth, the vendor has a right to inspect the inventory and to have access to it. This can create a problem if the vendor is out of stock and needs to "borrow" in order to fill another hospital's requirements. Fifth, establishing minimum and maximum inventory levels may be a point of disagreement. The vendor will want to maintain the minimum amount of inventory because of inventory carrying costs. Sixth, it is important to set a maximum time for the item to be maintained in consignment, keeping in mind shelf-life problems. Seventh, a clear rotation policy should be determined—for example, first in, first out. Finally, the method of invoicing for consignment inventory must be determined. Special inventory procedures may be necessary to verify usage. Will the vendor conduct the inventory or is the hospital responsible? Can the vendor's invoice be eliminated through the use of a special requisition, inventory control, and reporting procedures? These are most of the points that need to be considered before agreeing to consignment ordering.

AUTOMATED ORDERING SYSTEMS

During the past 15 years, the Bell System has developed and refined electronic order entry systems. One early system, called DataPhone, utilized key punched electronic data processing (EDP) cards to transmit orders. Today's systems utilize Touchtone and card dialer telephones, teletypewriter order entry, and teleprinters that provide for print-back of orders. These new order entry systems have made purchasing supplies as easy as touching a button.

In keeping with the developments of the Bell System, computer companies have developed new, sophisticated hardware and software packages to enable the vendor to accept this type of data entry. American Hospital Supply has refined its system, known as ASAP, and other national and local suppliers have also developed systems to accept electronic order entry. Colonial Hospital Supply, a Chicago-based firm, has developed a system known as TLC. Colonial's system is unique in that the computer's "human" voice, affectionately called Henrietta, talks you through order entry by repeating the item number and quantity ordered. Henrietta also informs you of the current stock availability before moving to the next item to be ordered. Other companies have developed systems that electronically transfer an image (copy) of the purchase order to the vendor within minutes.

Each of the systems described has advantages and limitations. Most claim to offer the opportunity to reduce ordering and delivery time. Adding a print-back unit reduces the clerical functions required to type orders. In many cases, these claims are true. Limitations include using the standard vendor print-back format, which is probably different from the hospital's standard purchase order format. In addition, the time saved in typing may be offset in identifying storeroom stock numbers and the department cost centers for which merchandise was ordered. Also, the number of copies provided through the print-back (most have a maximum of five parts) may not be sufficient to meet the hospital's purchase order distribution requirements.

The future of electronic devices as an aid to the procurement process appears to be unlimited. There seems to be little doubt that future systems will permit orders to be processed by the hospital's computer directly to the vendor's computer with minimal "human" intervention. The potentials of electronic order processing are limited only by operating costs and human acceptance of the electronic order processing concept.

Nevertheless, the practitioner must remember that these electronic devices are but tools to be used to improve some clerical efficiencies. Such devices will not automatically reduce your inventory or eliminate your back-order problems totally. The practitioner must utilize the data they provide to improve these two areas. Cost containment is something the practitioners, not the electronic devices, make happen.

SYSTEMS CONTRACTS

As a concept, systems contracting, on the one hand, has been hailed as one of the best cost containment ideas; and, on the other, maligned as one of the worst purchasing practices in use today. Despite this wide disparity of opinion, systems contracting (also referred to as prime vendor) is a concept that is and will continue to be a viable alternative for the practitioner.

Systems contracting is based upon the concept of purchasing a majority of a given product category, commodity, or classification from one primary vendor. As defined here, systems contracting does not suggest that *all,* but rather that *most,* items of a product category are purchased from one supplier. It is important that the practitioner understand that we are talking about a majority (51 percent plus) of and not an entire product category. This distinction is made because no one supplier can provide all of the products within a given category that the hospital requires. Thus, it is possible that a majority of a product category can be purchased from a single vendor with other vendors meeting the remainder of the hospital's requirements.

Product categories that easily lend themselves to system contracts include forms, housekeeping, laboratory, linens, medical/surgical, intravenous (IV) solutions, office supplies, pharmaceuticals, and radiology.

As indicated earlier, systems contracting has its advantages and disadvantages. Among the advantages are:

- The hospital can maximize its buying power by offering the vendor a large percentage of business for an extended period of time. Because the vendor recognizes that the receipt of this business is "guaranteed" for the specified period, distribution and administrative costs can be spread over a larger dollar volume of anticipated business, thus resulting in lowered unit costs to the hospital.

• Both the hospital and the vendor should be able to realize economies through the reduction of inventory. This advantage is based upon the premise that the hospital provides the vendor with specific information relative to order quantity and frequency for individual line items. Through a cooperative effort, the vendor should realize economies in purchasing and pass these economies along to the hospital. Further, economies by the hospital can also be improved through improved service, resulting in reductions in reorder points and safety stocks and thereby reducing inventory.

The single most often cited disadvantage is that systems contracting requires the hospital to give up the freedom to purchase competitively. Because of the impact that this position presents, it is important to examine its ramifications.

If we assume that systems contracting results in one vendor gaining a monopolistic position for a given commodity or classification, then the situation becomes acceptable if it results in (1) a pricing advantage to the hospital, (2) improved service, and (3) an agreement that is limited in time. The time limitation is important because it enables the hospital to terminate the agreement if the vendor cannot maintain the pricing and service commitments.

It is also important to recognize that competition is limited if the systems contract is entered into without the benefit of all vendors having the opportunity to bid for the contract. If competitive bidding is utilized to award the systems contract, then one would assume that the best "packaged" contract will be attained. That brings us to the next point to be clarified—the package.

Practitioners must recognize that with a systems contract, some individual line item prices may be higher than those currently being paid. However, when individual line items are taken in the aggregate, the net result should be lower total annual costs overall.

A systems contract should include the following basic components. First, the terms of the contract should be limited in time. Opinions on the duration of a systems contract vary from one to three years; two years appears to be an optimum period for both the vendor and the hospital.

Second, pricing should be based upon a specific percentage from the best quantity price. This pricing should apply regardless of quantities ordered on individual purchase orders.

Third, escalation limits should be determined for the second year of the contract. This most probably will require negotiation with the vendor, but is a necessity to prevent indiscriminate price increases.

Fourth, delivery and service standards should be clearly defined by the hospital and a penalty clause inserted in the contract. This penalty clause should allow the hospital to recoup the difference between the contract price and the price paid to another vendor who was able to meet the hospital's immediate requirement.

And fifth, a motivation percentage based upon total dollars should be included. This percentage should increase as the annualized dollars increase.

As a final comment, systems contracting is a viable alternative to be used by the practitioner. It is a sound concept that, if used properly, can result in cost savings to the hospital. Systems contracting requires open competitive bidding, aggressive negotiation, and persistence in accomplishing the objectives of lower total cost and improved service.

EXPEDITING

Any discussion of ordering systems requires inclusion of the expediting function (see Exhibit 5-3). As a legitimate part of the procurement cycle, expediting becomes necessary when back-orders of unknown duration exist, when an accelerated need for the item develops, and when the hospital is dependent upon the vendor's inventory in a stockless purchasing program.

Expediting programs can be either centralized or integrated. In a centralized program, one person or subsection of the purchasing department is solely responsible for the expediting function. This type of program offers several advantages: the need for fewer personnel; less expense; and a more concentrated effort. Its major drawback is the difficulty with communication and coordination between the buyer, expediter, and requesting department.

An integrated program is one where the buyer is responsible for placing the order and ensuring delivery. The advantage of an integrated program is that one individual is responsible for the order from placement to receipt. Its drawback is that it may require hiring additional buyers, thus incurring higher salary costs. The necessity for additional buyers results from the loss of time that should be devoted to prepurchasing and cost containment activities. For the smaller hospital, the integrated program will probably be essential because of the limitations of available resources and for practicality. The larger hospital should explore the potentials of a centralized program from the perspective of efficiency and consolidation of responsibility.

As a practical method, a personal approach utilizing telephone calls is usually more effective than the use of printed forms. The principal reason for the personal approach is that forms tend to be ignored, lost, or misplaced in someone's incoming basket. The personal approach also facilitates the main ingredient of an effective program, communication. The expediting process is really the art of persuasion. The expediter's primary objective is to persuade the vendor to process your hospital's order before those of other hospitals, and this requires good communication skills. The expediter who tends to use a heavy-handed, threatening

Exhibit 5-3 Expediting Procedure

```
                                                    PROCEDURE
                                                    MMPD-008
                                                    6/16/80


                        ST. FRANCIS HOSPITAL
                        BLUE ISLAND, ILLINOIS

                     MATERIEL MANAGEMENT DEPARTMENT
                        PURCHASING  DIVISION
                           EXPEDITING

                              POLICY
```

Purchasing is responsible for all expediting, follow up, handling
rejections, complaints, and returns concerning purchased equipment
and supplies.

```
                              PURPOSE
```

To ensure the timely flow of materiel required for the continued
operation of the hospital.

```
                             PROCEDURE
```

I. Routine Expediting

    A. On a daily basis, the expediter will review all open orders,
        after all the previous days receiving has been posted.

    B. Vendors are to be contacted by telephone and provided with all
        pertinent information regarding the open item(s). Note on the
        purchase order the date of the follow up, name of the person
        contacted, and the anticipated delivery date obtained.

    C. Contact the requesting department to advise them of the
        anticipated delivery time. If the requesting department
        cannot accept the anticipated delivery date, the order becomes
        a STAT order.

    D. If the vendor claims that the order has been delivered, a
        proof of delivery must be provided.

    E. If after two attempts, no delivery date is obtained or an
        anticipated delivery date is missed, the purchase order will
        be given to either the Purchasing Agent or Buyer for additional
        action.

II. STAT Expediting

    A. Any item that must be received in less than three (3) days
        is to be considered a STAT order.

    B. All STAT orders will be checked on a daily basis beginning
        with the day prior to the expected delivery date.

Exhibit 5-3 continued

C. If the vendor is unable to meet the delivery requirements, the expediter will:

    1. Seek an alternate source of supply, confirm price and availability, place a new order, and cancel the original order.

OR 2. Contact the requisitioner to determine if an acceptable substitute is available and place an order for the substitute.

D. Failure of a vendor to meet a STAT delivery date should be so noted in the vendor's completed file with a copy to either the Purchasing Agent or the buyer.

Director, Materiel Management

approach will be ineffective in the long run, whereas the expediter who motivates the vendor to make a real effort to meet the hospital's requirements will be more productive.

The development of an effective expediting program should involve the following.

- Know the vendor. Get to know the vendor's customer service personnel on a first-name basis. Promote an atmosphere of friendship and cooperation. Keep the names of contact personnel on the vendor card.

- Get help from receiving. Impress upon the receiving department the necessity for processing shipments and paperwork promptly.

- Know the method of shipment. Make a list of various shipping methods, the time frames involved, and the cost associated with each method.

- Think before you act. Always have all the associated paperwork for the order in front of you. Know what the delivery requirements of the ordering department are so that a decision can be made without a second or third call.

- Get all the facts. During the conversation make notes of when the order will be shipped, how it will be shipped, and whether it will be shipped partially or completely, and of the name of the individual making the promises. Keep all notes with the order for possible future reference.

- Check to see that promises are kept. Keep a "tickler" file to ensure that delivery has been made. If not, follow up immediately. Laxity on the part of the expediter tends to encourage late delivery by the vendor.

- Thank the vendor. When a vendor comes through, a "thank you" is always appreciated. Vendor relations tend to improve and future cooperation will be easier.

- Try to improve delivery requirements. Work with requisitioners on planning requirements in advance. Concentrate efforts on departments that consistently place STAT or rush orders.

- Select a good vendor. The time to reduce the probability of delivery problems is at the time of vendor selection. Remember, one quality of a good vendor is prompt delivery.

Chapter 6

Receiving

The final step in the procurement cycle is the receipt and taking formal possession of the merchandise ordered. Often dismissed as a routine clerical duty assigned to the storeroom, receiving is the final point in the procurement cycle at which mistakes can be detected and remedied. Errors by either the vendor or purchasing can be costly to the hospital if not detected when the merchandise arrives at the hospital receiving dock. The discussion that follows reviews the proper receiving procedure and the resolution of discrepancies.

RECEIVING PROCEDURE

Typical receiving procedures require that all or most of the following actions be completed. (An example of receiving procedure is shown in Appendix 6-A.)

1. Check and verify all packages and weights against the carrier's bill of lading.
2. Observe and record the condition of packing or other evidence of rough handling. With the carrier's representative present, quantify acceptance accordingly on the bill of lading.
3. Stamp all copies of the bill of lading with the date and stamp reading "Merchandise Received Subject to Inspection and Approval." Stamping the bill of lading with this type of statement protects the hospital in case of hidden damage to the contents within the package or carton.
4. Sign bill of lading with full name and retain one copy for record purposes.
5. Verify all merchandise received against the packing slip and the receiving copy of the purchase order. The receiving copy of the purchase order will be the primary source document for determining the correctness of an item.
6. Record discrepancies on the receiving report for action by purchasing and accounting.

7. Record receipt, either partial or complete, of merchandise on the receiving copies of the purchase order.
8. Deliver merchandise to proper ordering department.
9. Obtain the signature of the individual accepting delivery of the merchandise for the ordering department.
10. Process copies of the receiving report to purchasing and accounting.

DISCREPANCIES

As noted, undetected errors can be costly to the hospital if they are not identified during the receiving process. The following are typical examples of errors that can occur.

Short shipment. A short shipment occurs when the actual quantity received is less than the quantity shown on the vendor's packing slip. Note that the packing slip is the primary source document and not the purchase order. Partial shipments make the packing slip the primary document.

Overshipment. An overshipment occurs when the actual quantity received exceeds the quantity ordered on the purchase order.

Incorrect item. An incorrect item received is an item that does not match the description, catalog number, or quantity per ordering unit as described on the purchase order. This may also involve a substitute item shipped by the vendor without prior approval by the purchasing department.

Outdated items. This error occurs when a dated item is received that exceeds its original expiration date (normally imprinted on the package).

Damaged merchandise. This occurs when the external packing carton is received in damaged condition or when the merchandise inside the container sustains damage that renders the item unacceptable for its intended purpose. It should be noted that occasionally damage to the exterior of the shipping carton does not harm the merchandise inside. When this happens, it becomes a matter of judgment as to whether a claim for damages should be filed with the carrier or the vendor. The responsibility for processing claims for damage will depend upon when title of ownership passes to the hospital. A review of the discussion of FOB points in Chapter 1 should clarify this particular problem. Regardless of who processes the claim, it is important to keep the shipping carton, especially in claims of hidden damage. Responsibility for the damage usually rests with either the vendor or the carrier, and the shipping carton will be important in determining this responsibility.

Receipt of merchandise that was not ordered deserves special mention. Every day hospitals receive merchandise that was never ordered. When this type of situation occurs, the practitioner should make an effort to contact the vendor to arrange for the merchandise to be picked up; usually five working days are allowed. If, after the fifth working day, the vendor's arrangements have not been communicated to the purchasing department, the merchandise should be shipped to the vendor collect.

CHECKS AND BALANCES

The receiving process presents a potential for such control problems as delivery of merchandise to an incorrect department or processing receiving reports for merchandise ordered but never received. To preclude the possibility of any impropriety arising during the receiving process, practitioners should establish audit procedures to verify that routine procedures are being completed.

A typical receiving audit procedure requires that all of the following actions be completed.

1. Select five to ten recent purchase orders that include a balanced mix of recurring and nonrecurring items. At least one or two purchase orders should be for merchandise that could be subject to pilferage.
2. Verify that all of the steps included in the receiving procedure (described earlier in this chapter) are properly completed.
3. Verify that purchasing's and accounting's documents contain the same information.

Receiving procedures should be audited three or four times per year, and without advance notice to receiving personnel. This lack of advance notice will preclude the possibility of receiving personnel "preparing" for the audit. In conducting audit procedures, the practitioner should maintain a low profile. The purpose of the audit is to determine if the receiving department follows established procedure in inspecting and accounting for the goods it receives. Its purpose is not to cast a shadow of doubt over the people who are responsible for the receiving function.

Once the audit is completed, any discrepancies or procedural weaknesses that are discovered should be discussed with the individuals responsible. Any changes required or additional followup training that is deemed necessary should be completed as quickly as possible.

APPENDIX 6-A

ST. FRANCIS HOSPITAL	PROCEDURE
BLUE ISLAND, ILLINOIS	MMCSD-008
	8/23/79

MATERIEL MANAGEMENT DEPARTMENT
CENTRAL STORES DIVISION
GENERAL RECEIVING PROCEDURE

POLICY

All materiel ordered for use within the hospital must be received and inspected by Central Stores personnel.

PURPOSE

To provide for formal possession of ordered materiel and to ensure that this materiel conforms to the established standards of the hospital.

PROCEDURE

I. Upon delivery of materiel by a carrier, departmental personnel will, before taking formal possession, complete the following:

    A. Check and verify all packages and weights against the shipper's manifest.

    B. Observe and record condition of packing or other evidence of rough or faulty handling, with the carrier's representative present, prior to acceptance, qualifying acceptance accordingly on manifest. (See paragraph IX.)

    C. Stamp all copies of manifest with date and stamp reading "Merchandise Received Subject to Inspection and Approval."

    D. Sign manifest with full name and retain one copy for record purposes.

II. After formal possession, all materiel will be inspected and checked for accuracy.

    A. The packing slip will be located and a determination made of the hospital's purchase order number.

B. All merchandise received will be physically verified for accuracy and correctness against the packing slip and the receiving copy of the purchase order. *The receiving copy of the purchase order will be the primary source document to determine the correctness of an item.*

III. Partial receipt of an order.

A. All orders will be verified against the original receiving report and properly annotated at the bottom with the item number, date received, quantity received, quantity due, and initials of person who verified the order.

B. Copies of partial receiving report shall be distributed as follows:

(1) Purchasing—along with the manifest and packing slip
(2) Accounting

IV. Completed order with previous partial shipments.

A. When the balance of an order is received, the original receiving reports will be completed and distributed as detailed under paragraph V.

V. Completed order—one shipment.

A. All orders will be verified against the original receiving report and properly annotated at the bottom with the item number, date received, quantity received and initials of the person who verified the order.

B. Distribution of the completed receiving report shall be as follows:

(1) Receiving (canary)—to appropriate file
(2) Receiver—Accounts Payable (green)—to Accounting
(3) Receiver—Purchasing (pink)—to Purchasing

VI. The individual delivering materiel received will obtain a signature on the top copy at the time of delivery.

If no one is physically present to receive the materiel, the receiving report will be annotated to show time of delivery, where the materiel was left and initial of individual making delivery.

VII. Central Stores personnel are responsible to see that receiving reports are distributed to the appropriate departments by 4:00 P.M. daily.

VIII. Discrepancies.

A. *Short Shipments*—If during the physical verification process the actual quantity received is less than the quantity shown to be shipped on the packing slip, Central Stores personnel will attach a note to both the Purchasing and Accounting copies of the receiving report indicating that a shortage exists. The item number, quantity received and total amount of the shortage will be noted.

B. *Overshipments*—If during the physical verification process the actual quantity received is greater than the quantity ordered, Central Stores personnel will attach a note to both the Purchasing and Accounting copies of the receiving report indicating that an overage exists. The item number, quantity received and the total amount of the overshipment will be noted.

Only the amount ordered will be delivered to the ordering department. The amount of the overshipment will be retained until disposition has been decided by Purchasing.

C. *Incorrect Item*—If during the physical verification process the item received does not match the item ordered on the purchase order, Purchasing will be notified of the discrepancy with a note showing the purchase order number, item description of the item ordered and the description of the item received.

The merchandise received will be held in Central Stores until the discrepancy is resolved by Purchasing.

IX. Receipt of damaged goods.

A. If during the process of delivery, damage is noted to the shipping container, Central Stores personnel will:

(1) check to determine if there is only physical damage to the merchandise. If there is physical damage—refuse the item and note such damage on the manifest.

(2) If there appears to be no physical damage to the merchandise, accept delivery and note carton damage on the manifest.

B. If during the process of physical verification hidden damage to the merchandise is discovered:

(1) retain the shipping container;
(2) notify Purchasing immediately of the hidden damage;
(3) hold the item in Central Stores until the damage claim is resolved by Purchasing.

Director, Materiel Management

Chapter 7

Accounts Payable

The first six chapters of this text dealt with the techniques and problems associated with the procurement process. We now come to the area that is probably the least understood by many practitioners—accounts payable.

The culmination of the procurement cycle takes place in accounts payable. Purchasing provides for the acquisition portion of the cycle; receiving confirms that the materiel has been received in good order; and accounts payable provides for the financial process and control that ensure prompt, authorized, and accurate payment to the vendor. Mistakes or delays that occur in any portion of the procurement/receiving/accounts payable continuum can have an impact on the hospital's credit standing in the financial community. The more efficient the system, the greater the potential for a good credit standing. Therefore, it is important that the practitioner understand the accounts payable process.

SYSTEMS APPROACH TO DOCUMENTATION

In Chapter 1 it was noted that accounting should receive a copy of the purchase order and requisition to provide for proper invoice certification, payment, and voucher authorization. In Chapter 6 it was also noted that a copy of the partial/completed receiving report is sent to accounting to provide proper documentation of the receipt of the items ordered. All of the necessary paperwork is brought together in accounts payable for payment of the invoice. Sound simple? Well, it is a simple process—with a few subtleties that need to be clarified.

The systems approach to any procedure states that each portion of the system should complement the other portions of the total system. Thus, the accounts payable portion of the system should complement the purchase order system, and vice versa. Accounts payable, therefore, should maintain its copy of the open purchase orders in vendor sequence identical to purchasing's. Compatibility of open order filing systems is important to provide for joint, periodic review of the two files. A joint review will help to ensure that both departmental open order files are up to date and accurately reflect the financial commitments of the hospital. As a recommended routine, a joint review should be conducted semiannually.

To supplement the open order file, two additional files should be maintained: "Received—Not Billed," and "Billed—Not Received." Each file will contain purchase orders that lack a specific document, either an invoice or receiving report, necessary for further processing. These files should be reviewed periodically (once a week) to determine necessary followup actions either by accounting (invoice) or purchasing (receiving report).

Once all of the required documentation has been received and collated, the verification process can begin. Each line item on the purchase order and the invoice is verified for quantity ordered, received, and invoiced. Additionally, unit pricing and extended costs on the invoice are verified against what is shown on the purchase order. Transportation charges are also reviewed against the purchase order. However, this review of transportation charges by accounting is usually limited to verification of FOB points to determine if the hospital is responsible for payment of any freight charges that may be reflected on the invoice. When the hospital is responsible for freight charges, it is the practitioner's responsibility to obtain estimated freight charges that are as accurate as possible, and to reflect this estimate on the purchase order. In almost every instance in which the hospital is responsible for freight charges, the vendor should be requested to provide a copy of the freight bill as supportive documentation for charges on the invoice.

The next step is the calculation of any discounts for prompt payment. Finally, the invoice is coded for proper expense distribution to the ordering department. The entire paperwork package is sent to data processing for processing of the voucher. This systemized verification process takes place for every purchase order and invoice that is received by accounts payable. All things being equal, the vendor is paid on time and the procurement cycle is completed. Unfortunately, all things are not always equal and problems begin to arise.

PROBLEM SOLVING

When the human equation is involved in any specific systematic process, mistakes are going to happen. In the procurement continuum, unless an obvious accounting error is made, delays in the payables process are the fault of either the purchasing practitioner, the receiving department, or the vendor.

The following is a composite list of errors or reasons why accounts payable sends an invoice to purchasing for correction. Some of these errors may appear a bit ludicrous to the experienced practitioner, and they are. But even experienced practitioners have made them at one time or another.

- Ordering quantity and unit cost do not match. An example of this error is when the purchase order reflects an order quantity of 100 each and the unit cost is by case of 100. The vendor's invoice has one case at the correct case price.

  Probable cause: Most often this happens when a traveling requisition system is used. Order quantity is verified by the vendor, and the traveling requisition was not changed before the purchase order was typed.

  Solution: Clean up your act! Accuracy is important. Every transaction should be reviewed prior to having the purchase order typed. Clerk typists only type the information they receive. A change order is now required to make the purchase order and invoice agree before payment can be made.

- Quantity ordered and received do not match.

  Probable cause: Normally, this is the result of: (1) overage/shortage in shipment; or (2) change in quantity ordered to meet vendor minimum or case quantity. The latter usually occurs with orders that are mailed rather than telephoned to the vendor.

  Solution: (1) Overages and/or shortages must be resolved with the vendor. A change order or credit memorandum will be required, depending upon how the problem is resolved. (2) Vendor minimums should be noted on the vendor card. A change order is necessary for payment and probably was not prepared when purchasing was notified by the vendor.

- Product item number and description on the purchase order and invoice do not match.

  Probable cause: Either a substitution was made or the wrong item was shipped and received.

  Solution: Vendors should be required to have advance approval from purchasing for substitutions. If substitutions are approved, a change order should be prepared at the time of approval to reflect the change. When an incorrect item is shipped and received, a thorough review of proper receiving procedures should be conducted with receiving personnel.

- Unit pricing on the purchase order and the invoice do not match.

  Probable cause: This problem has a whole host of probable causes. Among them are wrong list price used, wrong discounts taken, and failure to note a recent price change.

  Solution: Pricing should always be confirmed with the vendor when the order is placed. Where discounts are in effect, the purchase order should always reflect the net pricing. The accounting clerk should not be expected to calculate discounts.

- FOB terms do not agree.

Probable cause: This is the main problem for accounting. It results from not clearly indicating FOB terms on the purchase order and accounting not clearly understanding what the terms mean.

Solution: Every purchase order should clearly state the FOB terms on its face. It is also a good idea to prepare a list clarifying these terms for accounting to use as a reference. Refer to Chapter 1 for clarification of FOB terminology.

- Cash terms/prompt payment discount.

  Probable cause: Confusion arises in accounting in determining when the discount period begins and ends (i.e., receipt of goods or invoice).

  Solution: Clarify with the vendor at the time of negotiation or order placement and clearly identify on the purchase order when the discount period begins. Time determination is purchasing's responsibility, not accounting's.

- Wrong account number used.

  Probable cause: Wrong account number was used by the ordering department on the purchase requisition.

  Solution: For some unexplained reason, accounting will hold invoices for payment when a wrong account number is identified on the purchase order for distribution purposes. Many accounting personnel believe it is purchasing's responsibility to review and correct wrong account numbers. It is, in fact, the responsibility of the ordering department to identify properly the account code to be charged. It is recommended that accounting and purchasing review proper financial distribution coding with those departments that are consistently incorrect.

- Invoice received with no purchase order written.

  Probable cause: In a majority of cases, either a physician, department head, or other employee of the hospital has exceeded his/her authority and purchased something without using the purchasing department. A second possible cause is the fraudulent invoice.

  Solution: When a physician or hospital employee exceeds his/her authority, this becomes a particularly difficult problem for the practitioner. Two courses of action are available. The first is to discuss the problem with the offending individual. Explain the need for proper procedure, and then write a purchase, after the fact, to process the invoice properly. The second course of action is to send the invoice to the offending party, advising that payment of the invoice is the offender's responsibility. Experience says that if the second course of action is taken, the offender will go to administration, apologize for the error and promise never to do it again, and eventually get off the hook. The end result is that purchasing will process the paperwork anyway. It should also be noted that the physician or employee is not the only offender here. The vendor is also at fault for not obtaining a purchase order number. New vendors will claim ignorance of proper purchasing procedure, saying they did not know a purchase order was needed or that the individual involved did not have the authority to place orders. Therefore, in addition to the solution described, the invoice should be returned to the vendor on the grounds that it cannot be identified against a properly authorized purchase order. This obviously will delay payment and show the vendor the consequences of failing to follow proper procedure. New practitioners should not be fooled by the pleas of ignorance by the vendor. Requiring a purchase order is a standard procedure in industry as well as in hospitals.

The second possible cause of the existence of a fraudulent invoice requires special handling. Over the past few years, fraudulent invoicing schemes have occurred in many major metropolitan areas. Such a scheme usually involves altering the name of a well-known corporation and sending an invoice for a related product or service. Telephone followup on such invoices usually is unproductive. Practitioners who encounter a possible fraudulent scheme are advised to: (1) contact the Better Business Bureau or local Chamber of Commerce to determine any knowledge that organization possesses concerning the company; (2) contact the local metropolitan or state hospital association to determine whether other hospitals have reported similar situations; (3) contact the local post office to communicate your suspicion (mail fraud may be involved); (4) do not pay the invoice, but retain it for future reference.

- Invoice received with an incorrect purchase order.

  Probable cause: Normally, this is the result of a clerical error by the vendor.

  Solution: When accounting cannot verify the appropriate purchase order number, the invoice should be sent to the practitioner. It is the practitioner's responsibility to contact the vendor and correct the mistake.

- Return material/credit memorandums. The complexities of this form (described in Chapter 1) present the potential for problems for both accounts payable and receiving. Most of these problems are based on a misunderstanding of the reason indicated for the initiation of the form, and so practitioners must make clear exactly what is occurring and what anticipated results or expectations are to be achieved through the use of this form.

  When the need arises for the use of a return material/credit memorandum (RM/CM), accounting should be immediately notified to withhold payment of the invoice until the proper paperwork has been completed. Most often, the use of this form will necessitate a credit to be issued by the vendor. It is the practitioner's responsibility to ensure that the amount of credit to be received by the hospital is properly reflected on the form.

When an RM/CM form is used for return of damaged or incorrect material, the result will probably be a reshipment of replacement material. This situation necessitates receiving being aware of the receipt of new material and accounting being aware of a vendor mistake that could lead to double billing. Therefore, the practitioner must make every effort to clarify the actions and expectations by all individuals concerned with the transaction.

CHECKS AND BALANCES

The separation of procurement and payment has evolved as business has become more complex and the use of credit has expanded. Years ago, when life was simple, cash was the normal medium for transacting business between buyer and seller. The advent of credit brought with it the need to separate the functions of procurement and payment. But there is a more fundamental reason for this separation, honesty. The separation of responsibility serves to secure the institution from the possibility of claims of and occurrences of collusion in an effort to defraud the institution. If the institution establishes realistic procedures for invoice payment, collusion can occur only when the individuals representing purchasing, accounting, and the vendor are involved. While the possibility that such a situation actually will occur may appear to be quite small, the need for a proper system of checks and balances remains. Thus, accounting rightfully is responsible for remaining a neutral party to ensure that propriety is maintained at the highest possible level.

RELATIONS WITH ACCOUNTING

In recognizing the need for checks and balances, it is also necessary to maintain an open, communicative relationship between accounting and purchasing. Both departments need to work together to solve problems and to ensure, to the maximum extent possible, that the institution's financial resources are utilized to their best advantage. Harmonious relations should be the norm, and not the exception. Accounting can be the strongest ally of purchasing in achieving many of purchasing's goals and objectives. Together, purchasing and accounting can maintain and improve the financial stability of the hospital.

Chapter 8

Pharmacy and Dietary Purchasing

True centralized purchasing should be the goal of every purchasing practitioner. But only a very few have successfully accomplished that objective. The reason for the lack of centralized purchasing rests primarily in the resistance provided by a hospital's chief pharmacist and chief dietitian. Specialization and education are the primary arguments that these two departments present in defense of their desire to retain their own purchasing operations. But if this is true, why not let the laboratory, maintenance, and all the other departments do their own purchasing? They also are specialists. Some pharmacists have even claimed that state law allows only pharmacists to purchase drugs. All of these claims are nothing but a smoke screen.

Admittedly, some pharmacists and dietitians are good purchasing practitioners—but unfortunately, many are not. The discussion that follows explains what is required for the purchasing practitioner to purchase both pharmaceuticals and food.

PROCUREMENT OF PHARMACEUTICALS

Quality, service, and price determination apply to pharmaceuticals just as they do to medical/surgical supplies, housekeeping supplies, and everything else procured for use within the hospital. There are, however, some special considerations that must be explained.

Quality determination is not the responsibility of the purchasing practitioner or the product utilization committee. Quality is the responsibility of the pharmacy department in conjunction with the therapeutics committee. To understand the reason for this specialized quality determination, one must understand what pharmaceuticals are. Pharmaceuticals are medicinal substances—any chemical compound or noninfectious biological substance utilized in the diagnosis, treatment, or prevention of an abnormal condition. By their very nature, quality determination of pharmaceuticals requires the specialized knowledge of the pharmacist and the medical staff. In the opinion of this author, quality determination by the pharmacist and therapeutics committee is a nonnegotiable point. The purchasing practitioner's responsibility is to procure the quality product specified, and to accept no substitutions unless they are expressly approved.

If there is no room for negotiation of quality, where do generics fit in? Generic equivalents have their place in the hospital pharmacy, provided they are properly tested in terms of their physical, chemical, and biological properties. It is important for the purchasing practitioner to understand that many "generic equivalents" are marketed without research or testing to substantiate their properties. The major pharmaceutical manufacturers have already expended time and money on research to substantiate their claims. Many generics are simply copies or products repackaged under another name. For these reasons, generic equivalents require proper testing and evaluation prior to their use in the hospital. Physicians do tend to prescribe brand name pharmaceuticals rather than generics. This practice should not preclude generic testing. Again, this is the responsibility of the pharmacist.

Some purchasing practitioners believe that purchasing pharmaceuticals is as easy as consulting the "yellow pages." This is an erroneous assumption on the practitioner's part. The Red Book is a good reference, but a reference only, just as the medical/surgical manufacturers' listings and the Thomas Register are good references.

By now you are probably thinking that you may as well purchase exactly what the pharmacist orders, with no questions asked. Right? Wrong! Purchasing and pharmacy have a joint responsibility to maintain high standards for pharmaceuticals. This goal can be achieved only through open, responsive, two-way communication. Like everything else, there has to be a reason for preferring one manufacturer over another. The purchasing practitioner has a right to receive a reasonable answer. Most pharmacists have high-quality standards. Yet, they too want to achieve cost containment without sacrificing quality. Open communication is the key element.

Where to purchase pharmaceuticals is a practical matter. Like medical/surgical supplies, pharmaceuticals can be purchased from either the manufacturer or the wholesaler. Ideally, dealing directly with the manufacturer is the best course of action. Like other supplies, some manufacturers sell only through wholesalers. Eli Lilly is a good example. Lilly will not sell directly to hospitals. Regardless of whether you deal with manufacturers or wholesalers, the standards for vendor performance should apply equally in this area. Practitioners should also recognize that, like manufacturers for other commodities, back orders will occur. Pharmaceutical back orders require some flexibility on the part of the practitioner. Purchasing from wholesalers, at a potentially higher price, should be routine when the need requires immediate delivery. In other words, despite the fact that an order may already have been placed with the manufacturer or another vendor under a specific contract, if an immediate need arises for the product, the practitioner should not hesitate to fill the temporary requirements from another vendor, even if this means paying a slightly higher price. This brings us to the next consideration.

Pharmaceuticals can, and should, be subjected to the same procedures of competitive bidding and negotiation as all other supplies. Whenever possible, purchasing practitioners should not be limited to brand name buying. Remembering that quality determination is a key essential in the purchasing process, the practitioner should work closely with the pharmacy in evaluating the bids received. Group purchasing is also an effective technique for pharmaceutical purchasing. However, before using group purchasing, product quality and compatibility should be thoroughly checked prior to commitment.

Hospital pharmaceutical bid specifications should include projected annual requirements, generic descriptions, packaging requirements, terms and conditions of purchase, and other applicable specifications. Vendors should be required to provide net pricing (rebates are a common practice among pharmaceutical manufacturers and should be avoided); bioavailability information, when requested by the hospital; source of raw dosage form; quality control documents relating to the batch supplied (if other than the specific manufacturer specified), including test results and certifications; all terms of delivery; and invoicing and payment terms. Whenever possible, bids should be awarded on an annual basis for the same reasons as noted in Chapter 4.

Finally, there is also an exception in receiving pharmaceuticals, and that exception is with narcotics and other controlled substances. Because of their nature and tight government controls, narcotics require special receiving procedures. First, the product should be shipped in sealed containers with the exterior label marked "Medical Supplies, Rush." This identification, or some other special identification, should be used to alert receiving to the contents.

Second, the receiving clerk should only open the container in the presence of a pharmacist. Both the receiving clerk and the pharmacist should check the item(s) together. This procedure is recommended in case of shortages in shipment or damage to the product that renders it unfit for use. Further, this procedure of using two people provides added assurances as to any claims involving damage or shortage.

Third, both the pharmacist and the receiving clerk should sign the receiving report as proof of delivery. Narcotics and other controlled substances are not items to be taken lightly. The use of the two-person system provides a backup or check and balance for both individuals. Violations of federal laws covering narcotics usually result in someone going to jail.

With the few exceptions noted, pharmaceutical purchasing is not unlike purchasing other specialized commodities. All that is really needed is open communication and some common sense.

PROCUREMENT FOR DIETARY

As with pharmaceutical purchasing, food purchasing traditionally has been excluded from most purchasing departments' responsibility, principally because food purchasing requires specialized training. As a purchasing practitioner, this author tends both to agree and to disagree with this proposition. In many hospitals, most food purchasing is done by a clerk, and not by the dietitian. The clerk merely orders what the dietitian specifies. In a majority of cases, the dietary clerk has had neither formal training in proper purchasing procedures nor specialized dietary training. Thus, it should be obvious that purchasing practitioners can develop the knowledge required to procure food. The discussion that follows will aid in the development of this knowledge.

Specifications

The foundation for food purchasing is the need for written specifications. As with other specialized purchases, specifications are necessary to describe the quality desired accurately. The purchasing practitioner would do well to form a committee to develop such specifications—a committee composed of the dietitian, the chef, the cafeteria supervisor, and the practitioner. The committee's primary purpose is to correlate diversified requirements in order to produce specifications that are acceptable to everyone involved in the various areas of the food service operation.

Every effort should be made by the committee to determine whether there are any government or commercial specifications available that are appropriate, either whole or in part, for use by the hospital. If these specifications can be utilized, they can save valuable time that can be devoted to product testing and research. At the very least, these specifications can provide a starting point for the hospital's specific requirements.

The committee's efforts initially should be aimed at high-dollar-volume items. Such items can be identified through ABC analysis (Chapter 10).

Finally, it is important to recognize that the written specifications will serve not only as bidding documents, but also to ensure correct delivery, production planning, and portion control.

For the purchasing practitioner, it is important to know the terminology of food purchasing in order to develop specifications that meet the hospital's requirements and to understand the needs of the dietary department.

Canned Products

Canned fruits and vegetables are an important part of dietary menu planning. They also offer a number of advantages for both dietary and purchasing, including:

- They lighten the work load in the kitchen.
- They eliminate waste.
- Selection can be made to suit the need for and the use of the product.
- Brand names or U.S. Department of Agriculture (USDA) grading will eliminate guesswork concerning product quality.
- The buyer has control of style, size, quality, and count to meet the specific purpose.
- Normally, they are available the year around.
- They provide for easy portion control.
- They provide for convenient storage.
- Quantity purchases can result in significant cost savings.
- They are usually less costly than fresh products.
- Dietetic canned fruits and vegetables are often available for specialized diets.

Purchasing canned fruits and vegetables is done by grades established by the USDA. Grading is the most important consideration to be given to canned products. Normally, three grades are established for most products:

1. US Grade A or Fancy. This is the highest quality determination. Products that meet this grade are selected as to size, color, and maturity.
2. US Grade B or Choice. These products are not as uniform in color, size, and maturity as Grade A, but will normally satisfy the dietitian's requirements for appearance.
3. US Grade C or Standard. This grade is not as carefully selected as the other two grades. It usually sells at a lower price, but contains the same nutritional value as those products in higher grades.

The purchasing practitioner should also be aware that many food purveyors sell grades by the color of the can label. A red label equates to Grade A, a blue label to Grade B, and a green or black label to Grade C. Sometimes label colors will vary by region or purveyor and the practitioner is advised to verify the relation of color to grade.

The second consideration regarding canned products is style. For many products, usually more than one style is available. For example, green beans can be either cut or sliced.

A third consideration is variety. Like style, there is usually more than one. For apples, it is the distinction among Jonathan, McIntosh, Delicious, Baldwin, etc.

The fourth consideration is count size, which refers to the quantity per container. Counts of 48 and 72 are specific examples. When purchasing by count size, it is advisable to break down unit cost into portion or each cost in order to determine the cost effectiveness of the various count sizes.

Count size brings us to the fifth consideration—the size of the container. Canned products are sold either by volume or weight in the same size container. As an illustration, a number 10 can will hold 14 ounces of liquid measure or 3 pounds of solid measure. When purchasing on the basis of container size, be sure to distinguish between liquid or volume measurements. And when purchasing soups, it is a good idea to distinguish between soups that are condensed and those that are ready to serve. Both can be purchased in the same size container.

The sixth and final consideration for canned products is syrup density. Peaches and pineapples are typical items that are packed in syrup. Syrup densities usually are limited to light, heavy, and extra heavy. When combined with count size and/or container size, the density of syrup can appreciably affect product cost on a per-portion basis.

Fresh Foods

The purchase of fresh foods is not unlike purchasing canned products. The following considerations apply to fresh foods.

As with canned products, grading is the first consideration. Fresh food grades are established by the USDA, state regulations, or the growers and packers. Grading may vary by commodity, and most often will conform to the grading standards noted for canned products: fancy, choice, or standard.

The second consideration for the practitioner to understand is variety, quality, and uses for the various fresh foods.

The third consideration is style of packaging. Fresh food is packed in one of three styles:

1. Jumbled. With this packing, there is no specific order or layering.
2. Rowed or numerical count. With this method, the product is graded and packed in rows and layers by specific count.
3. Filled and faced. This is a combination of the first two styles, with the top uniform and the bottom jumbled.

The style of packaging will influence the fourth consideration, which is the fill of the container. Containers are sold as heaped, level, or scant. Heaped refers to something that exceeds the upper part of the container, for instance, a bushel basket. Level refers to being filled to the top of the container, and no higher. Scant means something less than what the container is designed to hold. Because of the lack of quantity determination, scant is not recommended as a fill specification.

Type of container is the fifth consideration. Determination of crate, box, carton, sack, bushel, or basket will influence the quantity, style, and fill of the container, as well as the price to be paid.

The sixth consideration for fresh food is the purchase of product in season. Fresh food purchased out of season will be expensive, if it is available. Quality of product for out-of-season foods is also something that may be suspect, especially when purveyors offer exceptional bargains.

Finally, it is important for the purchasing practitioner to have the ability to check fresh food visually for quality. Quality determination can have an effect on the cost effectiveness of the product. This ability can be gained by visiting various markets in the company of the dietitian or chef. Visiting your local supermarket can also be beneficial. How to determine the quality of fresh foods is the type of knowledge that can only be acquired from hands-on experience. As a routine practice, fresh foods should be inspected at the time of delivery, and either accepted or rejected immediately.

Purchase Process

The dietary purchasing process is not dissimilar to other purchasing processes already described. There are, however, some special considerations that must be noted.

First, the purchasing practitioner should work closely with the dietitian on menu planning. It is advisable to limit the menu cycle to three months in order to quantify potential requirements. The practitioner should be prepared for last minute changes by the dietary department, and also for a lack of availability of the desired product.

Second, the practitioner should not be afraid to challenge the dietitian on grade specifications. Dietitians not only want to serve nutritional foods, but also foods that look appetizing once prepared. For this reason, fancy grades are often specified. Often a lesser grade (choice) will provide the same nutritional value as a fancy grade, and be difficult to distinguish from a fancy grade. The choice grade will also be less expensive from a unit cost perspective.

Challenging grade specifications is going to be an area of discord with the dietitian. It is a recognized fact that the appearance of a meal can influence a patient's decision to eat or reject the meal as presented. Thus, the more appetizing the food looks, the greater the possibility it will be consumed. However, it should also be recognized that most patients cannot determine the grade of food that is presented. What a patient will determine is how it tastes, and that is directly related to preparation and not to grade. Proper preparation and consistency of temperature will influence consumption more than will the use of a fancy versus a choice grade in many instances.

Intended use of the product will also influence grade selection. For instance, the use of.fancy style peas in the dining room can be a waste of money. Some fancy styles are made to be cooked once and served immediately. When subjected to the heat of a steam table after initial cooking, a fancy pea that starts out looking appetizing can, in a matter of minutes, become green mush. Fit the grade and style to the product's intended use.

Third, exercise good inventory control. Fresh food should be purchased to fill immediate needs only. Canned foods should be subjected to good stock rotation. Many foods are highly perishable or have a limited shelf life. Good inventory control can save money and ensure that the food products maintain their quality integrity.

Fourth, both dietary and purchasing should be involved in vendor selection and evaluation. One practice that is advisable in the selection process is a can opening—when a vendor is requested to bring in samples of a product or group of products to be evaluated for quality, consistency, and can count. Can openings are also appropriate when products are introduced into the market after harvest.

The fifth consideration is price determination. The conventional competitive bidding process normally applied is of relatively little value in dietary purchasing. Daily price fluctuations in the food commodity market, especially for fresh foods, is normal. It is not practical for the practitioner to seek competitive bids on a daily basis. Nor is it practical to expect a purveyor to hold firm prices for any lengthy time period, for example, six months. A practical compromise is necessary in the purchasing process. For fresh foods, such as meat, seafood, and poultry, weekly firm prices can be a reasonable expectation. For canned products, monthly firm pricing may be a reasonable expectation. Current market conditions (supply and demand) will influence any firm pricing arrangements. Thus, it is necessary to keep up to date on what is going on in the market relative to available supply and current demand. It is also advisable to utilize group purchasing arrangements whenever possible. Group purchasing can sometimes influence the duration of firm pricing for certain commodities such as bread, eggs, and dairy products.

The last special consideration should be the establishment of a quality assurance program. Such a program should include, at a minimum, the following:

• Orders should be processed by purchasing within a specified time frame.

• Deliveries should be made at the time specified.

• Back orders should be identified immediately (at the time of order). Use of alternative purveyors should be a matter of routine.

• Ordered products should be checked routinely for quality and count against written specifications. Substitutions should not be accepted unless specifically authorized in advance.

In addition to these components, pricing should be compared periodically with prices paid by schools or other hospitals that utilize similar products. Comparisons should also be made in regard to purveyor performance. Unsatisfactory performance warrants the same actions normally applied to vendors of other commodities.

Chapter 9

Contract Services

The tremendous growth of the service industry during the late 1960s has made contracting for services one of the fastest growing elements of hospital purchasing. Virtually every major service provided within a hospital can now be performed by an outside service contractor. With this growth have come the problems of dealing with service contracts. There has never been a clear-cut established procedure in this regard, nor any set format for contracts or terms and conditions that specifically relate to service contracts. For this reason, hospital purchasing practitioners have relied on techniques basic to the procurement of supplies and equipment, and expanded these techniques to meet their needs for service contracting. (See Exhibit 9-1.) The discussion that follows attempts to clarify many of the common problems associated with contract services.

CLASSIFICATION

Contract services are divided into three classifications: professional, personnel, and facilities and equipment. Professional services in a hospital include consulting, data processing, and legal services, and physician services in the emergency room, radiology, and laboratory. Among personnel services are food, vending machines, and health services. The facilities and equipment classifications include housekeeping, security, and equipment maintenance.

In many hospitals, professional and personnel service classifications have not been included in the scope of the purchasing practitioner. The rapid growth and acceptance of the materiel management concept is changing this situation. Inroads are now being made to include purchasing in acquiring personnel services as well as facilities and equipment services. Similar inroads have not been as successful regarding professional service contracts. The exclusion of purchasing from this area has been justified by the "nature" of these contracts, which may be valid

Exhibit 9-1 Sample Procedure Policy

ST. FRANCIS HOSPITAL   POLICY
BLUE ISLAND,ILLINOIS   MM-004
                                        1/15/80
MATERIEL MANAGEMENT DEPARTMENT

CONTRACTS AND AGREEMENTS

POLICY

The Materiel Management Department will develop guidelines and format
for entering into all contracts and agreements in reference to purchase
commitments for supplies, equipment, and equipment services.

PURPOSE

To assure the proper development, approval, and documentation of all
contracts and commitments of the hospital in reference to supplies,
equipment, and equipment services.

PROCEDURE

1. The Director, Materiel Management or Purchasing Agent shall initiate
    all negotiations for all contracts for the hospital.

2. The following items should be considered in the development of such
    contracts:
    A. Length of contract.
    B. Enumeration of services purchased.
    C. Payment terms.
    D. Insurance and indemnity notification clause.
    E. Assignment and governing law reference.
    F. Transportation charges.
    G. Terms of cancellation.

3. All contracts and commitments for services are to be initiated
    through the normal hospital purchasing process. Therefore, a
    purchase order number is assigned to each contract.

4. The cost of providing the service must be a budgeted item.

5. Unbudgeted items must be approved by administration.

6. All contracts and long term agreements must be approved and signed
    by the Executive Director.

Director, Materiel Management

when the purchasing practitioner has minimal experience. However, experienced practitioners can assist administration in the contract definition, statement of expected performance, and protection afforded to the hospital in terms of liability, that is, insurance, etc.

TYPES OF CONTRACTS

The two basic types of service contracts are time and materials, and fixed price. With a time and materials contract, the contractor bills the hospital on the basis of total man-hours supplied, supplies consumed, and a reasonable profit. Time and materials contracts generally possess three major drawbacks: (1) high administrative costs; (2) the tendency for cost growth; and (3) difficulties in auditing allowable costs. As a general rule, time and materials contracts should be used only when it is impossible either to define the task desired or to measure satisfactory performance.

The fixed price service contract is the preferred alternative to time and materials. This contract is applicable to service contracts when it is possible to define the services to be purchased in quantitative terms and quantitatively to measure acceptance of the product or results of the service performed.

PURCHASING METHOD

The first step in the procurement process is to evaluate the need for a service contract. Most often department managers who desire the service contract believe they have done an adequate job of evaluating the need. Additional review by the practitioner is viewed as unnecessary and a waste of time. Despite this attitude, the practitioner should take the time to make an independent, objective analysis of the existing, or apparently existing, need.

The second step is to define clearly the scope of the service to be provided. This is the joint responsibility of the department manager and the practitioner.

For equipment service contracts, the practitioner should undertake discussions with the maintenance/biomedical maintenance supervisor. These discussions should center around reviewing current in-house capabilities and exploring the possible upgrading of the in-house staff.

When personnel services are involved, similar discussions should be undertaken with the personnel manager and administrator to review in-house capabilities.

If it is determined that the service cannot be performed in house, a buying team should be organized, comprised of the requesting department manager, the controller, and the practitioner. The team's objective should be to arrive at a contract that is acceptable to all departments involved and to ensure that proper controls and accountability are firmly established.

The team should explore the market of potential contractors to determine if more than one contractor is able to provide the desired service. If more than one contractor is available, the competitive bidding process should be set in motion. Where only one bidder prevails, the team should prepare for the negotiation process. The procedures for both competitive bidding and negotiation detailed in Chapter 4 should be used as a guide. Regardless of which procedure is utilized, the team concept should prevail in the final decision-making process. The award of these types of contracts is too important to be left to one individual.

At this juncture, it is important to note some of the problems that can be anticipated when competitive bidding is possible. Some department managers— laboratory, maintenance, and radiology, in particular—are going to complain about allowing a contractor other than the manufacturer to work on their equipment. In some cases, their concern may be justified. However, this problem can be lessened with pre-qualification of the vendor's reputation and capability to provide the desired services prior to inclusion on the bid list. It should also be clearly proved that the manufacturer can provide superior service at the proposed cost. Often this is not the case.

It should also be noted that the lowest bidder may not necessarily provide the best service. Once all of the bids have been received, a thorough review of the lowest bidding vendor should be undertaken to guard against misinterpretations. Should a problem surface, the next lowest bidder should be interviewed, and so on until the award is finally determined.

Finally, every effort should be made to sign a contract that includes all of the terms and conditions that the team feels are necessary to protect the rights of the hospital. Remember, standard vendor contracts afford maximum protection for the vendor and little, if any, protection for the hospital. Negotiation is the key to obtaining the desired services.

CONTROLLING

Akin to the purchasing process is the need for centralized control of all new and existing contracts. It is not unusual to find existing service contracts being maintained by a number of different departments throughout the hospital. The responsibility for controlling service contracts rightfully lies within the scope of the purchasing department. This responsibility should encompass all aspects of contract award and administration.

DOCUMENTATION

Supportive documentation is undoubtedly the weakest area in most hospital service contract programs. It has achieved this dubious distinction for two fundamental reasons: decentralization of control and inattention. For the purchasing practitioner, centralization of responsibility for controlling contract services brings with it the added responsibility to develop an internal control system to monitor contractor performance and resolve the inattentiveness problem. The discussion that follows should prove valuable in identifying and rectifying some of the typical problems associated with supportive documentation requirements and the establishment of proper procedure.

EQUIPMENT SERVICE CONTRACTS

The film processor in radiology has failed and a service call is placed to the contractor by a radiology technician on the day shift. The unit is repaired late the same afternoon, and an invoice is mailed to the hospital for parts used in completing the repairs. Accounting wants to know if the invoice is correct and requests authorization for payment. The chief technician was out that day and the corresponding service ticket cannot be located. None of the other technicians know exactly what work was performed. The chief technician authorizes payment to the contractor despite the fact that the invoice cannot be verified.

This brief scenario is typical of hundreds of similar situations that occur on a daily basis in hospitals all over the country. At best, this scenario is a sad, but true, commentary on the need for sound documentation procedures for service contracts in hospitals.

A good program begins by clearly establishing the responsibility for contracting the vendor. In most hospitals, the user is allowed to place the initial call. The rationale behind this method is that the user can clearly identify and explain the problem to the contractor. Technical questions can be asked and answered with the potential of solving the problem over the telephone. This method also assumes that the problem may involve the use of an incorrect procedure. If the problem is mechanical, the contractor should be able to bring the potentially necessary parts when the service visit is made. Users believe that this procedure tends to improve communication and reduce equipment downtime. As far as the user is concerned, it is the best procedure.

The alternative to the user placing the call is to require the user to notify purchasing, and purchasing, in turn, notifies the contractor. For the purchasing practitioner, this appears to be the best method because purchasing will not be aware that service is needed. User opinion of this procedure is characteristically unfavorable. The major user arguments against this procedure are that purchasing: (1) does not understand the technical aspects of the equipment; (2) tends to misinform the contractor of the problem; and (3) cannot answer the contractor's questions, thus resulting in the necessity for a return call to the user and wasted time. As a practical matter, the user's arguments are true in a majority of hospitals.

To purchasing practitioners who disagree with these arguments and demand that all service calls be placed by purchasing, let us address some key questions. Does purchasing know the technicalities of every piece of hospital equipment? Can purchasing respond to technical questions of the contractor? Does purchasing know the proper procedures for use of the equipment? The answers to these questions are no. It should be obvious that the user is much more knowledgeable concerning the equipment than the practitioner is. If the user's arguments are true, how does purchasing maintain control? The answer lies in compromise. Purchasing should retain control of service calls for typewriters, calculators, copy machines, and other types of office equipment. User calls should be authorized for other equipment on a case-by-case determination by the practitioner, provided that the user is willing to follow established procedures.

When user calls are determined to be the best procedure, the practitioner should create a contract call register. This call register, to be completed by the person placing the call, should contain:

- call number (beginning at one and continuing sequentially throughout the year)

- name of person placing the call

- serial number or other equipment identification

- date and time of call

- nature of the problem

- anticipated response time by the contractor

The call register will at least substantiate the fact the call was made, provide a basis for establishing the validity of need, and identify the person who initiated the call.

In conjunction with the call register, the contractor should have a list of individuals authorized to place service calls. The contractor should also be required to use the call number on all subsequent service tickets and invoices. Authorizing specific individuals to place calls will provide some control within the user department and, it is hoped, reduce unnecessary calls. Requiring call numbers on service tickets and invoices will prove useful for audit purposes. Both procedures should be clarified with the contractor at the time of contract   award.

The second step in establishing good control is to require all service technicians to sign into and out of purchasing. Other arrangements will be necessary for nights, weekends, and holidays. This procedure raises problems akin to those associated with vendor representatives wandering throughout the hospital. But it also provides purchasing with the knowledge that a service call was made.

The third step is to require that a copy of all service tickets be given to purchasing when the service call is completed. Every equipment service contractor should be required to provide the following information on the service ticket:

- serial number of the equipment repaired

- model number

- a clear statement of what was repaired

- a complete listing of all parts used and their associated costs

- total man-hours involved with the repair

- travel time (if it is part of the contract and the hospital is paying for it)

The need for this information will become apparent later in this chapter.

Closely associated with obtaining service tickets is being able to read them. It seems that service representatives take the same handwriting course that physicians do. Both groups are known to have handwriting styles that are almost illegible and impossible to decipher. Improving handwriting may be improbable, but not impossible, to accomplish. One tactic that gets results is to read the service ticket and ask the technician to explain what has been written. As with sales representatives, time is money to the service technician. Threatening not to pay the invoice until the service ticket is legible is also a good idea. After a couple of delays, service technicians begin to get the idea and many will take the extra few minutes necessary to get it right the first time.

The next item to be addressed is recording and utilizing the information on the service ticket. This step requires centralizing all of the relevant data for each piece of equipment. The question arises as to who should keep the data—purchasing or maintenance? As a practical matter, maintenance (or biomedical maintenance) should maintain the data on all equipment except office equipment. Purchasing should maintain the data on all office equipment. As a part of the procedure, purchasing should record only the total costs for parts and labor and forward the ticket to maintenance for posting to a maintenance record.

Maintenance should keep a centralized record for every piece of equipment regardless of who repairs or maintains it. This centralized record should contain information relative to:

- equipment description

- model and serial number

- date received

- unit cost

- length of warranty

- vendor and manufacturer

- number of service calls and the exact nature of each call

- amount and type of each part used

- man-hours expended and their associated costs

- an up-to-date summary of total service costs

Why record information on work performed by an outside contractor? There are three central reasons. The first is that should a piece of equipment fail and cause physical harm to either an employee or patient, the entire history of that piece of equipment may be required to support the hospital's case if litigation is started against the hospital and the contractor. Realistically, whether the work is performed by an outside contractor or in-house personnel, this type of record should be maintained.

The second reason is that at some point, the equipment will require replacement. If there is one claim that is made by the user to justify replacement, it is excessive downtime and maintenance costs. Without complete maintenance records to support these claims, the decision-making process is hindered by lack of specific information.

The final reason is the renewal of the contract. Contractors continue to increase the costs associated with the contract on the basis of equipment age, inflation, and rising labor costs. For the practitioner, a review of the historical data should be made prior to renegotiation to determine the validity of the contractor's claims.

The final step in the overall program involves payment of the invoice. For supplies and equipment, receiving reports are a matter of routine to substantiate proof of delivery and to authorize payment of the invoice. Service contracts do not readily lend themselves to the use of receiving reports and, therefore, require special handling procedures to verify invoices.

Routinely, invoices for service contracts should be reviewed and approved by both purchasing and maintenance. Both departments should compare the invoice with their respective records to ensure that the invoice accurately reflects the information contained on the original service ticket. When or if a discrepancy is discovered, purchasing should be responsible to resolve these discrepancies.

FACILITY CONTRACTS

Facility contracts, for such services as laundry, housekeeping, and security, also require documentation to support the costs incurred. Whenever possible, this documentation should be quantified. For example, laundry service can be verified by having a hospital employee verify all weights at the time of delivery.

Contracts for housekeeping, security, and similar services are not as easy to quantify and, therefore, require some subjectivism in evaluating costs. Because of the wide variety of the possible contracts of this nature, there are no clear-cut methods to quantify these costs.

ADVANCE PAYMENT CONTRACTS

Service contracts, specifically fixed price contracts, may require advance payment for services to be performed at a later date. Many preventive maintenance contracts fall into this category. Whenever possible, advance payment contracts should be avoided. If they cannot, payments should be negotiated on a monthly or quarterly basis—never on a semiannual or annual basis. The reason for this recommendation is that the hospital is paying for a service that conceivably it might never receive. It also means that the contractor is using the hospital's money for an extended period of time. This same money could be working for the hospital.

Where advance payments are required, the next billing should not be made by accounting until the work performed in the preceding period is verified. Again, service tickets should be used for this verification process.

DEALING WITH THE PHANTOM CONTRACTOR

For some reason, hospitals allow some contractors to perform their preventive maintenance or other maintenance responsibility at night when staffing is minimal. Contracts for anesthesia machines and pest control are typical examples. These phantom contractors enter the hospital, perform their necessary service, and disappear back into the night. For practitioners with this problem, it is strongly suggested that the practice be discontinued and all work be required to be done during normal operating hours. Now surgery and anesthesia undoubtedly will raise a fuss about the disruption of service that will cost the hospital valuable income. And employees, and perhaps the patients, are going to complain about the odor from the pest control sprays. So be prepared. The fact is that the hospital is already spending a lot of money for these services and has a right to know that they are being performed to its satisfaction. Further, these types of services can be scheduled far enough in advance to keep disruption of services and potential discomfort to a minimum. Creativity, cooperation, and understanding are the keys to success. The alternative may be paying for services that cannot be verified and that will cost the hospital more money than will any disruption of service.

Chapter 10

Inventory Management

The era of cost containment has brought with it the increased requirement for improved inventory control procedures. Under the materiel management concept, supplies are controlled from purchase through their final return to the environment. This chapter concentrates on inventory management for supplies under the control of the storeroom and/or central supply. The techniques described can also be applied to inventories in dietary, pharmacy, maintenance, and other departments that consume or store large amounts of "unofficial" inventory.

RESPONSIBILITY FOR INVENTORY MANAGEMENT

Regardless of whether or not a hospital has established the materiel management concept, one individual should be assigned the responsibility for inventory management. In the small hospital, this should be the highest purchasing practitioner. In medium and large hospitals, inventory management responsibility can be delegated to the storeroom manager or supervisor. But whenever possible, this responsibility should be delegated to someone other than the purchasing practitioner. Why? Good inventory management requires (1) a tremendous amount of time and energy, (2) constant vigilance for changes in usage and ordering patterns by using departments, and (3) changes in pricing that will significantly alter the value of the inventory. Inventory management is too important to be approached on a hit-or-miss basis, especially when hospitals are being asked to do more with less or limited resources. Inventory management presents a basic and cost-effective method of controlling rising hospital costs. As the term purchasing practitioner relates to a specialist, the term inventory practitioner should relate to a specialist in inventory management.

STORES CATALOG

The development of a stores catalog is the first step toward implementing an inventory management program. Although catalogs have been criticized for being too expensive to develop and maintain properly, a good catalog is as necessary for the storeroom as it is for the hospital's vendors. Can you imagine ordering supplies from a vendor without knowing whether the vendor stocks the item? Well, that is the first reason for having a stores catalog—to provide an accurate listing of the materiel maintained in the storeroom. The second reason is that a catalog provides a centralized listing to assist the hospital staff in the proper identification and requisition of material in regard to both quantity and quality. Again, try to order material from a vendor without knowing the product number and ordering unit and see how far you get (let alone what you receive). Third, a catalog, properly constructed, can contribute to the standardization of materiel within the hospital. Just as the vendor offers a variety of sizes and styles, so can the storeroom. Fourth, and finally, a catalog provides organization of the inventory, and this should result in better control with greater accuracy in maintaining proper stock levels. Thus, the development of a catalog leads to consolidation and accuracy of the materiel maintained in the storeroom.

The development of a catalog begins by taking an inventory of the storeroom to evolve accurate descriptions of those items that are already in stock. This step can often be accomplished simultaneously with a physical count inventory, thus accomplishing two objectives at the same time. During the inventory, you will want to obtain specific information relative to description, product number, quantity per ordering unit, and quantity of issuing unit if different from the ordering unit (i.e., ordering unit is "case;" issuing unit is "each").

The second step is the classification or categorization of the materiel. The classification can be as broad as medical/surgical, housekeeping, and office supplies, or as narrow as catheters, needles/syringes, or dressings. It is often advisable to clarify with accounting how the inventory dollars are carried on the hospital ledgers. More often than not, broad terms are used (e.g., medical/surgical) by accounting. When this is the case, you may want to develop specific subclassifications within these areas. For example, within the medical/surgical inventory, subclassifications for sutures, needles/syringes, and catheters can be utilized. Another method for broad term inventory classes is to list all of the items within a class alphabetically. Care must be taken not to be overly specific and thus detract from the usefulness of the catalog. Logic and practicality are the key words in catalog development. One of the reasons for a catalog is to provide the hospital staff with a useful tool to order supplies from the storeroom, so keep it simple.

The third step is to assign an alphabetical or numerical identifier to each classification. For example, if you decide to alphabetize within the broad category of medical/surgical supplies, "MA" can be used to identify medical/surgical (M) and then those items whose descriptions begin with the letter "A" (MA-001 applicators, cotton tipped, 3 inch). If a numerical indicator is preferred, a two-digit code should be satisfactory, that is, 01 representing medical/surgical supplies. It should also be noted that if a computerized inventory is planned, a numerical indicator is preferred to an alphabetical indicator.

Maintaining continuity of supplies within each classification is a must. For example, catheters should be classified together by type and then by size. Every effort should be made to develop a short, thorough, understandable, and accepted description for each item. This includes size, color, and a standard ordering unit. Whenever possible, generic descriptions should be used rather than specific manufacturers' identities. For example, the description "Tape, Zonas, 1 inch" refers to a specific manufacturer's tape, in this case J & J's. A better generic description is "Tape, adhesive, 1 inch." Utilization of the generic allows changes in suppliers to be made without extensive changes in the catalog.

After the classification is completed, a numerical code is assigned to each individual item within a category. The numerical code assignments can range from a two- to six-digit code. Normally, a four-digit code will be adequate. Sufficient numerical spacing should be used to allow for additions to the inventory. This procedure should be followed throughout the entire catalog development process. See Table 10-1 for a sample page of a stores catalog.

Once the catalog is completed, it may be necessary to revise ordering forms to facilitate departmental ordering by using the proper catalog number. Although you can expect some resistance from the hospital staff, insist on using the stock numbers for ordering. Such resistance can be reduced by conducting an in-service seminar to explain the change in procedure, how the catalog is organized, and the benefits to be derived from its use. Copies of the catalog should be distributed to all departments that order supplies from the storeroom. Consider using a looseleaf binder that will permit revisions and updating. A requisition schedule (if included) will contribute to an even distribution of the storeroom workload. Including hours of operation and other requisition information will also prove beneficial to everyone concerned with the use of the catalog.

Finally, the question of unit costs must be addressed. Many practitioners believe that the inclusion of unit costs is unnecessary and creates an additional burden because of the need for continued revision. Admittedly, constant revision will be a problem. Other practitioners feel that their inclusion will influence the hospital staff to become more conscious of costs and, therefore, to order smaller quantities that will adequately meet its immediate operating needs. Both arguments hold much merit. Inclusion of unit prices will, understandably, become a matter of individual choice. This author has developed catalogs both with and without unit prices. Inclusion of unit prices has raised the level of cost consciousness, and considerably improved the standardization process and cost reduction attitude within the hospital. However, the lack of unit prices in the other catalog did not

Table 10-1 Sample Catalog Page

Code Number	Description of Product	Unit of Issue	Unit Cost
AP - 75	Pencils, #2-2/4—gold sabre	12/bx	.96
AP - 80	Pencils, black paper wrapped, marking	each	.38
AP - 85	Pencils, red paper wrapped, marking	each	.24
AP - 90	Pencils, red verithin—Eagle	each	.21
AP - 95	Pockets, hinged 4×6—Acme	each	.15
AP - 100	Pockets, hinged 5×8—Acme	each	.25
AP - 105	Preservers, negative—10×12	500/bx	18.56
AP - 110	Preservers, negative—14×17	each	.07
AP - 115	Preservers, negative—14×17, prenumbered	200/bx	50.47
AP - 116	Protectors, sheet, 8½×11 B4-913	50/bx	4.00
AP - 120			
AP - 125			
AP - 130			
AP - 135			
AP - 140			
AR - 01	Ribbon for Terminet 300, AT-120 Blk.	each	3.25
AR - 02	Ribbon for Terminet 30, TN-30 Blk.	2/pkg.	16.00
AR - 05	Ribbon, printing calculator #E201	each	2.25
AR - 10	Reinforcements, gummed—Dennison 9/16	box	.15
AR - 15	Ribbon, typewriter, IBM, black general purpose #1136136	each	2.39
AR - 16	Ribbon, IBM Exec. Carbon Cartridge #1136182	each	1.13
AR - 17	Ribbon, IBM Selectric Fabric Ribbon #1136138	each	2.39
AR - 18	Ribbon, IBM Tech III Carbon Cartr. #1136391	each	7.36
AR - 19			
AR - 20	Ribbon, Olivetti ED. II, nylon red/blk. T-30	each	2.25
AR - 25	Ribbon, typewriter, blk. (Olympia-Underwood)	each	2.00

inhibit the level of cost consciousness and standardization. What it did was lengthen the time required to attain the degree of cost consciousness that was sought. Unit pricing in a storeroom catalog can be beneficial, if a proper perspective is maintained as to how unit costs are going to be used.

DETERMINING WHAT BELONGS IN INVENTORY

Many inventory practitioners believe that certain basic criteria must be established in order to determine whether an item will or will not be maintained in the inventory. Exhibit 10-1 illustrates some of the criteria used by inventory managers across the country. These criteria are all valid to those who use them, and reflect an effort to simplify the decision-making process. There are, however, two other criteria that are more meaningful to this process. They are that (1) there must be

Exhibit 10-1 Criteria for Inventory Control

---

1. Time and extent of probable use
2. Storage costs
3. Obsolescence
4. Shrinkage
5. Transportation costs
6. Investment costs
7. Cost to purchase
8. Quantity price differential
9. Market conditions and price trends
10. Time required for delivery
11. Availability of a substitute
12. Cash flow
13. Alternative investment potential

---

available space, and (2) it must be more economical to maintain an item in inventory than to purchase it on demand.

Many hospitals today face a critical shortage of available central storage space. This lack of space is usually the one criterion that dictates what will and will not be maintained in the inventory. While we all would like to have unlimited space in which to store and control items such as x-ray film, laboratory supplies, and dietary nonfoods, it is not always possible. Discussions with our colleagues over the past few years have revealed that the lack of available space is a problem for small and large hospitals from coast to coast. In Chapter 12 the problem of efficient space utilization is discussed in greater detail. For now, suffice it to say that unless your hospital has unlimited space available, the space required to store any item will become a major criterion in the decision-making process.

The second point, that it must be more economical to maintain an item in inventory than to purchase on demand, can also be as meaningful as the available space criterion. Before we explore the economics of inventories, it is important to establish why we have them. The primary functions of an inventory are twofold: (1) to provide maximum supply service consistent with maximum efficiency and optimum inventory investment; and (2) to provide a cushion between the forecasted and actual demand for a materiel. The goal of any inventory investment should be to support the attainment of the hospital's primary objective (patient care) with the optimum investment in inventory. Optimum inventory investment should not be confused with minimum inventory investment. Optimum investment may or may not be a minimum investment, depending upon various factors. These include the number of patients, patient mix (medical versus surgical), type of services provided, and location in relation to suppliers. Inventory investments are especially important to hospitals since operating funds are usually limited. The funds that are used for inventory are also the same funds required for salaries, capital equipment, and general operating expenses. Every inventory practitioner must strive to operate with optimum inventories, provided that, in doing so, the achievement of other objectives (patient care) is not jeopardized.

The second function, to serve as a cushion between forecasted and actual demand, is largely created by the inability to forecast accurately. This inability to forecast is also created by the same factors mentioned previously (number of patients, patient mix, etc.). All businesses and hospitals have difficulty managing their inventories. Yet no business can operate without one. Inventories protect against unforeseen failures in supply, increased demand, or unanticipated delays in delivery. Thus, inventory is not a luxury, but a necessity to achieve the objective of patient care.

Returning to the economics of inventory, inventory practitioners must maintain objectivity in this decision-making process. The following are questions that need to be asked concerning any item:

1. What are the anticipated annual usage and associated costs?
2. What is the intended use of the item?
3. Is the item applicable for use by more than one department?
4. What are the consequences of not having the item available (both real and perceived)?
5. What are the economic consequences of allowing the individual department to control the inventory of this item (both real and perceived)?

Questions 1, 4, and 5 can be measured through the use of quantitative methods described later in this chapter. Questions 2 and 3 require objective answers and analysis. Question 3 usually invokes another question: Are items used exclusively in the emergency room, intensive care units, and surgery special cases? Again, an objective judgment is required by the inventory practitioner. In the opinion of this author, the answer is a definite *maybe!* The subjective influences exerted by members of the respective nursing staffs can often be excessive. As a general guide, subject the item to the normal rationale established for inventory items. If the item is marginal, inventory the item at minimal investment levels, and let time become the determining factor.

INVENTORY RECORDKEEPING SYSTEMS

During the past five years, the subject of inventory recordkeeping systems has received considerable attention. Manual perpetual inventory recordkeeping systems have been considered too expensive to operate, inefficient, and perpetually wrong. To many inventory practitioners, computerized perpetual inventory systems have been the wave of the future, and the future is now! While the future may be now, the need for some type of inventory recordkeeping is very real. Large hospitals have computers available for inventory recordkeeping, but small hospitals need access to computers as well. Both manual and computerized recordkeeping systems have their place in hospital inventory management practices. In fact, the best computerized systems have been those developed from good manual systems.

Any discussion of inventory recordkeeping must begin by defining the term "perpetual inventory." In a recordkeeping sense, a perpetual inventory is a continuous account of the incoming supplies (receipt), outgoing supplies (issues), and the balance on hand. At practically any moment in time, the perpetual inventory records should give the actual balance on hand and the activity for any particular inventory item.

In utilizing this system, there is no need to segregate stock because the control is maintained with records for each item, and all transactions are posted to the record. Each transaction must be substantiated by some form of documentation, such as a receiving report or requisition. The inventory record should always reflect the balance on hand and on order, so that it is possible to calculate the value of the stock at any time.

Why is it necessary to calculate "on order?" Normally, inventory practitioners believe that calculating the on-hand balance is sufficient to determine the value of the inventory. In 98 percent of the cases, the on-hand balance will satisfy the accounting requirements. However, if you remember the earlier discussion on FOB points, you must recognize that any item that is FOB shipping point becomes the property of the hospital at the time of shipment. When this is the case, the value of that stock should be reflected in the inventory record even though it has not been formally received by the hospital. While this procedure is correct in the strictest accounting sense, many inventory practitioners show only the on-hand balance because they do not know when the item was shipped. Inventory practitioners should clarify this procedure with the hospital controller to ensure its correctness and necessity.

Inventory practitioners must recognize that any perpetual inventory system, whether manual or computerized, will be expensive to operate. While the cost of a perpetual inventory system is easily justified for valuable items subject to loss from pilferage, the need for a total system can often be completely justified on the basis of total dollars expended through the storeroom.

MANUAL SYSTEMS

As previously noted, manual perpetual inventory systems have come under fire because of the expense involved and their lack of accuracy. At a seminar a few years ago, this author listened to a recognized authority in materiel management, the president of a large medical/surgical supply corporation, condemn the manual system and extoll the value of a computerized system both as to speed and to accuracy. The remarks were logical. However, one point that was not made is that any system, manual or computerized, is only as good as the people who operate it. The old adage of "garbage in, garbage out" applies equally to both types of recordkeeping systems. Years of personal experience with both have shown that often it is not the system design that is faulty, it is the people who operate the system who are. Therefore, any system requires complete training of the operating personnel.

Traditionally, practitioners have also believed that a manual system requires some type of cardex system, such as those available from Acme Visible or Victor Visible. A cardex system involves an investment in expensive file cabinets and the hiring of an inventory control clerk to operate it. All documentations (receiving reports and requisitions) are given to the clerk for posting to the perpetual inventory cards. This type of system is expensive and potentially inefficient in its daily operation.

At St. Francis Hospital, Blue Island, Illinois, a simple manual system has been designed that requires no special cabinets or additional personnel. A recent audit of the system reflected a 99 percent accuracy level. This system utilizes three cards: a stock record card (Exhibit 10-2), an on-order card (Exhibit 10-3), and a traveling requisition (Exhibit 1-2, see Chapter 1). Both the stock record card and the on-order card are maintained with the merchandise. Requisitions are posted to the stock record card when the merchandise is removed from the shelf. The department, date of issue, quantity issued, and balance on hand are entered at the time of issue. When the balance on hand reaches the reorder point, the order card is annotated with the balance on hand and the date the order is initiated. It is then given to the storeroom supervisor, who initiates the traveling requisition to purchasing. The order card is held until the traveling requisition is returned from purchasing, when the vendor and purchase order number are entered. The order card is then placed in a file box in the receiving section. When the item is received, the order card is annotated with the date and quantity received and placed with the item. When the stock is placed on the shelf, the receipt is posted to the stock control card and the cards are clipped together. No one individual is responsible for any part of the system. Because the storeroom clerks rotate between receiving and issuing duties, they understand all aspects of the system and the importance of completing each part. This system is inexpensive, easy to use, and accurate. It is both informational and people oriented, and the people make the system work.

Associated with the manual system is a complementary back-order system. When a requisitioned item is not available for immediate issue, the item is marked as a back order on the department's original requisition. A back-ordered item slip (Exhibit 10-4) is created and attached to the stock record card. Only one back order per department per item is honored by the storeroom. This action is necessary to

Exhibit 10-2 Stock Record Card

ITEM				STOCK NO.	MAX.
DISP. UNIT					MIN.

NO. RECEIVED	NO. ON HAND	ISSUED TO DEPT.	DATE OF ISSUE	NO. ISSUED	BALANCE
		TURN	CARD	OVER	

Exhibit 10-3 On-Order Card

ITEM				STOCK No.	MAX.
DISP. UNIT					MIN.

No. ON HAND	DATE ORDERED	No. ORDERED	VENDOR	DATE RECEIVED	No. RECEIVED	BACK ORDER

Exhibit 10-4 Back-ordered Item Slip

```
┌──────────────────────────────────────────────────────────┐
│                                                            │
│                    BACK ORDER ITEM                         │
│                                                            │
│                                                            │
│     DATE:_____         │
│                                                            │
│     DEPT:_____         │
│                                                            │
│     CODE: _____         │
│                                                            │
│     UNIT OF ISSUE: _____         │
│                                                            │
│     QUANTITY:_____         │
│                                                            │
│     UNIT COST: _____         │
│                                                            │
│     A  H  M&S  TOTAL:_____         │
│                                                            │
│     DATE FILLED: _____         │
│                                                            │
│     BY: _____         │
│                                                            │
│     REC'D. BY: _____         │
│                                                            │
│     21-04                                                  │
│                                                            │
└──────────────────────────────────────────────────────────┘
```

prevent needless overstocking by the departments and is cost effective in aiding in the reduction in unofficial inventory.

When an item is back-ordered, storeroom personnel initiate an immediate followup to purchasing (Exhibit 10-5) indicating that an out-of-stock condition exists. This form triggers two actions. First, purchasing immediately expedites the order according to normal procedures (assuming, of course, that it has not already done so from a previous request). And second, the storeroom supervisor reviews the usage history to determine if a revision is required to either the reorder point, safety stock, or economic order quantity (EOQ) for the item. Many times this action identifies vendor problems not previously recognized by the purchasing department and appropriate action can be taken to rectify them. Or a change in usage is noted that was not previously discerned.

Exhibit 10-5 Followup Request

```
PJS                                  DATE_____
                        ME
     Stock # _____
PLEASE EXPEDITE SHIPMENT

VENDOR_____ PO _____

REASON:_____

      _____

      _____

ACTION TAKEN: _____

      _____

      _____

21-02
```

COMPUTERIZED SYSTEMS

Automation of inventory recordkeeping is a concept whose time has arrived. The need for timely, accurate, and organized data for controlling and monitoring supply costs increases with each passing day. The pressures of cost containment and potential government intervention only add requirements for automated recordkeeping.

Automated inventory control, for both official and unofficial inventory, centers primarily around computers that are neither complex nor awe inspiring to those practitioners who understand the basic fundamentals of their operation. Designed to duplicate, amplify, and extend certain powers of the human intellect, computers have become more than mere machines that perform mathematical operations. Today's computers offer speed, total recall, and accuracy through their ability to process information by receiving, storing, operating on, and outputting data acting on predetermined instructions programmed into the computer's memory.

Virtually all control functions of inventory management can be performed by the computer, including forecasting, planning, and purchasing. It is important for the practitioner to perform a thorough investigation into the possible applications with a clear determination of cost versus benefits. The economic justification can be simplified if the benefits are defined in terms of basic central objectives, which normally include:

- reducing total inventory

- improving control of inventoried items

- automating clerical tasks

- providing management with useful information

- providing the desired degree of supply services

The computer can assist in achievement of these objectives if the applications are properly designed and implemented.

System Design

The foundation of any system design is the database. The database should be developed with care, so that all present and future needs are anticipated. The ability to program future applications and the beneficial life of these applications are critically dependent upon the database structure. The normal approach to computer programming is to define the applications first, and then design the database to support these applications. But while this is the most acceptable method, many programmers have chosen to build the database prior to defining the applications.

Assuming that system applications are completed first, the information required for each application should be listed with the application. Once all of the required information has been determined, the next step is to compare the requirements for each application to determine the common elements necessary for inclusion in the database. For inventory management, the following items are generally required to build the database:

- item number—a unique number for each item or catalog number

- item description—a brief, clear description of the item (This field is usually limited to a maximum number of characters and requires careful consideration.)

- unit description—the unit of measure by which the item is issued from inventory

- unit cost—the cost associated with the unit description by which the item is issued

- reorder point—minimum quantity level in issue units

- reorder quantity—the normal quantity ordered in issuing units

- item location—the location of the item in storage

- item type—the item classification of either A, B, or C

The following information can be developed for inclusion in the database at the discretion of the practitioner, depending upon the amount of available record storage, and application to current and future requirements:

- last purchase vendor number—normally the same vendor number assigned by accounting, which will become the basis for an accounts payable interface if such a program is to be developed

- number of times ordered in last year

- last time purchased (month and year)

- last time issued (month and year)

- current year-to-date receipts—in both quantity and dollar value formats

- current year-to-date issues—in both quantity and dollar value formats

Data Collection and Dissemination

The method of data collection and dissemination is critical to the usefulness of the information contained in the reports. The time interval between when a specific transaction occurs and when a decision is made will influence the reliability of the information. Both collection and dissemination are highly dependent upon the capabilities of the hardware in use.

Data collection can be accomplished through the use of either of two methods: punched cards, or direct input via a remote terminal (cathode-ray tube, or CRT). The use of punched cards requires manual preparation of the data by either an inventory control clerk or data processing. The conversion of data from the original documentation (for example, purchase order, issue requisition, receiving report) requires an extensive verification process prior to transmission to the computer. Input via a remote terminal (CRT) is a faster method of data conversion and verification because built-in editing criteria within the computer's software require immediate correction prior to input acceptance.

The dissemination of input data will depend upon the method of collection. Use of punched cards normally results in periodic reporting that schedules output reports on a fixed-time and fixed-date basis. Periodic reporting permits efficient scheduling and greater utilization of the central computer processing hardware. Periodic reporting does, however, restrict the flexibility of information reporting because it is not always possible to change the scheduled output time. If periodic reporting is utilized, the practitioner should seek to obtain the most frequent schedule possible. If daily reporting is not possible, two or three processing periods per week should be sought as a minimum.

The use of a remote CRT normally is associated with a real-time system. Real-time systems require that a response to an input transaction be recorded and processed, and the output from the processing be available in time to effect the next transaction. Real-time systems require expensive hardware and software capabilities to accommodate large amounts of data.

Ideally, a real-time system is the most desirable from a decision-making, information-gathering, and output-reporting perspective. Realistically, many hospitals will apply this type of capability to other applications within the hospital over the inventory system.

Input

Automated inventory systems require the same information processing as a manual system: purchases, receipts, issues, and adjustments. Normally, these transactions can be processed together or in any combination. The following sequential processing is the norm with automated systems:

1. All input is sorted by item number and transaction type, and is edited (verified) with the inventory master file.
2. Purchases are processed first, updating the quantity ordered, cost, and dates. A record should also be created for purchase control.
3. Receipts are processed next. The receipt is edited with the purchase record. The quantity received will reduce the on-order amounts, and increase the on-hand quantities and associated dollar values.
4. Adjustments (price changes, on-hand quantity changes other than issues, unit of measure changes, etc.) are the third type of transaction processed.
5. Issues are the last transaction processed for inventory items. The inventory is reduced by the quantity and associated dollar value.

Output Reports

The resulting reports for input processing should be developed to meet the informational requirements of the practitioner. The type of reporting will depend upon the frequency with which the information is desired. Output records are usually processed on a daily/weekly, monthly, and annual schedule.

Daily/Weekly Reports

The following reports are normally generated during the routine processing cycle.

Inventory transaction edit. This report identifies those transactions presented for processing and rejected. The reason for the rejection is usually identified so that correction can be accomplished prior to the next processing cycle. Table 10-2 is an example of this report.

Transaction register. This report summarizes all of the transactions, by inventory number, that have occurred during the processing cycle. Table 10-3 is an example.

Inventory requirements listing. This report (Table 10-4) reflects all of the items that have reached the reorder point. Note that the example provided includes items already on order and their expected delivery dates. These items are included to provide the practitioner with a notification that order expediting may be necessary to prevent a stock-out situation.

Inventory open order report. Closely associated with the requirements listing, this report (Table 10-5) provides a listing of open orders that are past the expected delivery date. Again, this report is used to initiate expediting procedures.

Inventory cost comparison report. This report is generated from receipts that are processed, and it provides information relative to price changes. Table 10-6 shows a listing of all receipts processed. This report can be modified to be generated only when a price change occurs.

Monthly Reports

Immediately after the last scheduled daily/weekly processing cycle of the month, a summary should be made of all transactions processed during the month. The following reports should be created.

Monthly transaction register. This report will summarize all of the daily/weekly transaction registers. In addition, it should also reflect the closing balances for all items in the inventory even though they may not have been specifically affected by the daily/weekly processing. This procedure is required to provide one single listing for reference purposes.

Department issue summary. This report provides a summary of items issued and their associated values on a monthly plus year-to-date basis. Two formats are recommended. First, a report by department (Table 10-7) that reflects issues to each specific department should be given to department heads for budgetary purposes. The second format (Table 10-8) is a summary listing, by department, that reflects total dollars for the current month and year to date.

Table 10-2 Inventory Transaction Edit

DATE   013080

INVENTORY TRANSACTION EDIT

RECORD TYPE	TRANS CODE	INV CODE	ITEM NUMBER	DATE	QTY	TOTAL COST	VENDOR CODE	ERROR MESSAGE
1 ORDER	53998	141	AO143	012480	30	2.00	01928	INVALID ITEM NUMBER
2 RECEIPT	53881	141	AO225	012480	10	0.58	11257	INVALID P.O. NUMBER
5 ADJ CANCEL	24310	141	AB023	012480	5	5.27	02359	INVALID P.O. NUMBER
8 ISSUE	62201	143	MS124	012480	2	1.13		INVALID ITEM NUMBER

TOTAL ERROR MESSAGES   04

Table 10-3 Daily Transaction Register

DATE   013080

DAILY TRANSACTION REGISTER

VENDOR	P.O.NR.	DATE	TYPE	TRANSACTION QTY	COST	VALUE	DISP COST	BALANCE O/H	VALUE	ON ORDER
MD 24	TONGUE DEPRESSOR ADULT STERILE									
			OPEN					10	27.00	
21943	54067	010980	ORD	20	3.00	60.00	2.70AV			20
21943	54067	011380	REC	15	3.00	45.00	2.88AV	25	72.00	5
21943	54067	011780	REC	2	3.00	6.00	2.89AV	27	78.00	3
4521		011980	ISS	4	2.89	11.56	2.89AV	23	66.44	
5021		011980	ISS	4	2.89	11.56	2.89AV	19	54.88	
			BAL**					19	54.88**	3
MP 319	EYE PADS, DISPOSABLE									
			OPEN					120	432.00	
5021		011980	ISS	3	3.60	10.80	3.60AV	117	421.20	
			BAL**				3.60AV	117	421.10**	

Table 10-4 Inventory Requirements Listing

DATE 013080

INVENTORY REQUIREMENTS LISTING

CODE	DESCRIPTION	UNIT	QTY O/H	EOQ	ROP	QTY ORDERED	DATE ORDERED	DATE TO BE RECEIVED
MA002	ADAPTER 18G LUER STUB	BX	0	3	1			
MA003	ADAPTER 23G LUER STUB	BX	0	3	3	3	011280	011980
MB024	URINE BAG, PED STERILE	BX	1	4	2	4	011280	012380
MB035	BLADE SURG #11	BX	1	3	2			
MB036	BLADE SURG #12	BX	1	2	1			
MC073	CATH FOLEY 5CC 18FR	CS	2	3	2			

Table 10-5 Inventory Open Order Report

DATE 013080

INVENTORY OPEN ORDER REPORT

CODE	DESCRIPTION	QTY	UNIT	DATE ORDERED	DATE TO BE RECEIVED	PO NR	VENDOR	
MD024	TONGUE DEPRESSORS ADULT	3	BX	011080	012480	54063	21943	AMERICAN HOSP SUP.
MS304	SUTURE 4-0 BLK #1677H	4	BX	011080	012280	54089	22877	BURROWS CO.
MA003	ADAPTER 23G LUER STUB	3	BX	011280	011980	54100	21943	AMERICAN HOSP SUP
MB024	URINE BAG, PED STERILE	4	CS	011280	012380	54102	23998	COLONIAL HOSP SUP

Table 10-6 Inventory Cost Comparison Report

DATE 013080

INVENTORY COST COMPARISON REPORT

CODE	PREVIOUS QUANTITY	QUANTITY RECEIVED	CURRENT QUANTITY	QUANTITY BACK ORDERED	PREVIOUS COST	PURCHASE COST	AVERAGE COST	PERCENTAGE CHANGE
AF110		2	2		10.40	10.40	10.40	0.00 %
AF112		2	2		8.93	8.93	8.93	0.00 %
AF220	1	10	11	10	9.50	9.50	9.50	0.00 %
HA115	1	4	5		65.00	66.68	66.34	2.06 %
MC023		2	2		19.50	20.00	20.00	2.56 %

Table 10-7 Department Issue Summary

Stock Number	Description	Unit Order	Price	Quantity	Current Month Total	Ytd. Total Quantity	Ytd. Total Amount
A0165	Labels Addressograph White	roll 1M	6.30			2	12.60
AC337	Paper 3 In. Scratch Roll	each	.60			1	.60
AC377	Patient Name Cards Hollister	pkg. 144	1.35	2	2.70	3	4.05
AC380	Pencils 2 Lead	each	.05			6	.30
AC405	Pens Fine Ball Point Red	each	.10	6	.60	18	1.80
AC410	Pens Fine Ball Point Black	each	.10	24	2.40	60	6.00
AC435	Ribbon Royal Black Typing	each	1.33			1	1.33
AC500	Tape ½ Scotch	roll	.57			2	1.14
	Total Items Requisitioned			32	5.70	93	27.82
D0150	Straws Disp. Plastic Flex	box 400	1.21	1	1.21	1	1.21
	Total Items Requisitioned			1	1.21	1	1.21
HC120	Deodorant Airwick Solid in Color Dispenser	each	.96			4	3.84
HC130	Deodorant Kleenaseptic Surface Spray	each	1.91	2	3.82	2	3.82
HC135	Deodorant Virotec Spray Disinfectant	each	2.14			4	8.56
H0221	Soap Dial 1 Ounce Bar	pkg. 20	1.56	1	1.56	2	3.12
HC270	Toilet Tissue	case 96	23.61			1	23.61
	Total Items Requisitioned					13	42.95
L0200	Albustix	bottle	4.85	3	5.38	3	14.55
	Total Items Requisitioned					3	14.55

M0130	Bandaid Plastic Strips ¾ × 3	box 100	1.99	1	1.99	2	3.68
M1780	Safety Pins Medium	pkg. 144	.62			2	1.24
	Total Items Requisitioned			1	1.99	4	4.92
PC175	Fluid Balance Sheet	pad 100	2.01			1	2.01
P0180	Fluid Chart, Intake & Output	pad 100	.83	2	1.66	4	3.32
PC232	Kardex Cards 5×8 Nursing Top	each	.03			150	4.50
PC347	Nursing Service Report 8½×14	pad 100	4.72			1	4.72
PC351	Nursing Discharge Summary Sheet	pad 100	1.91			3	5.73
P0465	Preoperative Check List	pad 100	1.78			1	1.78
P0500	Supply Room Order Requisition 5½×8½	pad 100	2.96			1	2.96
P0532	Team Leader Daily Report Sheets	pad 100	1.44			2	2.88
	Total Items Requisitioned			2	1.66	163	27.90
	Total Items Requisitioned			39	15.94	277	119.35

Table 10-8 Year-to-Date Department Issue Summary

Dept. 998 Hospital Summary

Supply Items Requisitioned and Charged Off

Stock Number	Description	Unit Order	Price	Quantity	Current Month Total	Ytd. Total Quantity	Ytd. Total Amount
M1187	Gloves Size 7½ Surgical Sterile	case 4	37.13	2	74.26	11	631.63
M1186	Gloves Size 8 Surgical Sterile	case 14	67.13	2	134.26	11	691.63
M1189	Gloves Clarion Surgical Sterile Size 8½	case 14	39.00	1	39.00	1	39.00
M1192	Gloves Size 6½ Surgical Sterile	box 4	33.84	1	33.84	6	343.49
M1194	Gowns, Disposable Converter	case 50	27.95			3	83.85
M1200	Incontinent Pads 23×36	case	17.50	47	822.50	122	2,135.00
M1203	Infant Suction Set Sterile	case 50	36.15			1	36.15
M1280	Invalid Cushions Inflatable	case 12	13.50	2	27.00	4	54.00
M1285	Irrigation Bulb Syringes Asepto Disp.	case 50	33.32			1	33.32
M1290	Irrigation Sets Disp.	case 20	23.75	7	166.25	19	451.25
M1300	Kerlix Fluffs Medium	case 60	33.75	3	109.23	9	311.73
M1302	Kerlix Sponges Sterile 55	case 60	65.65	7	459.55	23	1,509.95
M1310	Kerlix Roll Sterile	case 10	56.36			2	112.72
M1335	Kleenex/Scottie Tissues	each	.31	27	8.37	61	18.91
M1340	Kleenex/Scottie Tissues	case 36	11.02	20	220.40	61	672.22
M1345	Kling Bandage Roll 2> Bulk	case 96	13.18	1	13.18	2	26.36
M1350	Kling Bandage, Roll 3 Inch Bulk	case 96	20.49	4	20.49	2	41.64
M1355	Kling Bandage Roll 4 In Bulk	case 96	24.05			1	24.05
M1360	Kling Bandage Roll 6 In Bulk	case 48	18.78	1	18.78	1	18.78
M1365	Kling Bandage, Roll 2 Inch Sterile	case 96	22.81	1	22.81	1	22.81
M1370	Kling Bandage Roll 3 In. Sterile	case 96	30.03	3	90.09	3	90.09
M1375	Kling Bandage Roll 4> Sterile	case 96	36.50			3	106.86
M1380	Kling Bandage Roll 6> Sterile	case	24.63	1	24.63	2	49.26
M1385	Kotex Maternity Pads	case 60	11.87	13	154.31	38	451.06
M1387	Lavage Gastric Kit, Adult	each	3.00	1	3.00	1	3.00

Item	Description	Unit					
M1388	Lavage Gastric Kit, Pediatric	each	3.00	1	3.00	1	3.00
M1390	Lemun Glycerine Swabs	box 25	2.14	24	51.36	62	132.60
M1410	Levine Stomach Tubes #18 Fr.	case 50	23.20			1	23.20
M1412	Levine Stomach Tubes Sump 18 Fr	case 50	45.00	1	45.00	3	131.00
M1430	Lubricating Jelly 2 Grm	carton	6.16	3	18.48	6	36.96
M1432	Lubricant 5 Gram Packet	box 48	9.25			2	18.50
M1434	Lubricant, 5 Ounce Tube	box 12	4.68	9	42.12	24	112.32
M1435	Lumbar Puncture Tray Disp	case 20	132.41	1	132.41	2	246.51
M1445	Mask Aseptex Surgical	case 12	89.64	1	89.64	1	89.64
M1450	Mask Filtron Surgical	case 30	39.50	8	316.00	27	1,066.50
M1453	Maternity Care Kits	case 6	34.62	18	623.16	50	1,731.00
M1455	Medicine Cups Disp 1 Oz	pkg 100	.48	494	237.12	1602	768.96
M1460	Medicine Cups Glass	each	.19			12	2.28
M1465	Medicut Cannula 16 Gal	box 50	37.00			1	37.00
M1470	Medicut Cannula 18 Gal	box 50	41.50	1	41.50	6	249.00
M1475	Microdon Dressings 2×6	box 25	9.83	1	9.83	2	19.66
M1480	Microdon Dressings, 2>×8>	box 25	11.54	1	11.54	3	35.10
M1490	Modess Pads Vending	case 25	21.36	1	21.36	3	64.08
M1492	Montgomery Strips	box	13.99	2	27.98	3	41.97
M1500	Myelogram Tray Disp	case 10	94.00	1	94.00	2	188.00
M1505	Nail Polish Remover Delph	box 100	2.71	5	13.55	11	28.43

Annual Reports

Most hospitals require a physical inventory at the close of the fiscal year. The following reports are used in conjunction with the annual inventory or whenever an inventory is required.

Physical inventory worksheet. This report is a listing (Table 10-9) of all inventory items in location and the item number sequence. The worksheet is used to record the actual count and to update any pricing changes that may have to be made accurately to reflect the value of the inventory. Items are listed by location to ensure that each location in the storeroom is counted.

Physical inventory comparison report. Once the physical inventory worksheets are completed and verified, the items are matched with the inventory master file and a listing is prepared that indicates the actual physical count versus the inventory system quantities and their differences. As Table 10-10 shows, the current value of the physical inventory is calculated and compared with the system value. Once this listing is verified, the inventory master file should be updated with the physical count and value. Normal processing can begin again.

Special Reports

To complete the list of available reports, the computerized system should have the capability to produce the stores catalog, bin labels, vendor analysis, nonissue listing, and an ABC analysis report. Tables 10-11 through 10-13 are samples of these reports. Frequency of preparation is a decision for the practitioner. Vendor performance and the nonissue listing should be requested at least quarterly for review and analysis.

Table 10-9 Physical Inventory Worksheet

PHYSICAL INVENTORY WORKSHEET

DATE 122779

LOC.	CODE	ITEM DESCRIPTION	UNIT	QUANTITY	COST
24	MG035	GAUZE, SALVAGE,PLAIN 1/2 IN	JAR		
24	MG040	GAUZE, SALVAGE,PLAIN 1 IN	JAR		
24	MG045	GAUZE, SALVAGE, IODOFORM 1/4 IN	JAR		
24	MG100	GAUZE, PACKING, 2 IN X 100 YDS	ROLL		
24	MM050	MASK, FACE, J&J 4239	BOX		
24	MN025	NEEDLE, HYPO. 18G X 1 1/2 IN DISP	BOX 100		
24	MN030	NEEDLE, HYPO. 20G X 1 1/2 IN DISP	BOX 100		
24	MN035	NEEDLE, HYPO. 21G X 1 1/2 IN DISP	BOX 100		
24	MN040	NEEDLE, HYPO. 23G X 1 1/2 IN DISP	BOX 100		
24	MN045	NEEDLE, HYPO. 25G X 5/8 IN DISP	BOX 100		
24	MN050	NEEDLE, BIOP. 16G X 3 IN	EACH		

INITIAL _____

Table 10-10 Physical Inventory Comparison Report

DATE 010280

PHYSICAL INVENTORY COMPARISON REPORT

CODE	ITEM DESCRIPTION	UNIT	COST	QUANTITIES			DOLLAR	
				PHY. INV.	DATA INV.	DIFF.	PHY. VALUE	DIFF.
MG035	GAUZE,SALVAGE,PLAIN 1/2 IN	JAR	3.50	10	10	0	35.00	.00
MG040	GAUZE,SALVAGE,PLAIN 1 IN	JAR	3.65	8	10	2-	29.20	7.30-
MG045	GAUZE,SALVAGE,IODOFORM 1/4 IN	JAR	7.50	12	12	0	90.00	.00
MG100	GAUZE,PACKING 2 IN 100 YDS	ROLL	19.50	1	1	0	19.50	.00
MM050	MASK, FACE, J&J 4239	BOX	15.00	10	9	1	150.00	15.00
MM025	NEEDLE,HYPO,18G X 1 1/2 IN	BOX	7.50	20	20	0	150.00	.00
MN030	NEEDLE,HYPO,20G X 1 1/2 IN	BOX	7.50	2	2	0	15.00	.00
MN035	NEEDLE,HYPO,21G X 1 1/2 IN	BOX	7.50	12	11	1-	90.00	7.50-
MN040	NEEDLE,HYPO,23G X 1 1/2 IN	BOX	7.50	20	10	10	150.00	75.00
MN045	NEEDLE,HYPO,25G X 5/8 IN	BOX	7.50	15	15	0	112.50	.00
MN050	NEEDLE, BIOP, 16G X 3 IN	EACH	13.00	2	2	0	26.00	.00
	TOTAL			112	102	10	867.20	75.20

Table 10-11 Computerized Bin Labels

LOC. 24 M-0204 CS/72 BANDAGE, WEBRIL 3 IN. REORDER POINT 10 REORDER QTY 5		LOC. 24 M-0205 CS/36 BANDAGE, WEBRIL 6 IN. REORDER POINT 10 REORDER QTY 5
LOC. 24 M-0210 CS/96 BANDAGE, KLING 2 IN. REORDER POINT 10 REORDER QTY 5		LOC. 24 M-0220 CS/96 BANDAGE, KLING 4 IN. REORDER POINT 10 REORDER QTY 5
LOC. 24 M-0223 CS/96 BANDAGE, KLING 6 IN REORDER POINT 10 REORDER QTY 5		LOC. 24 M-0235 BX/50 BLADES, RAZOR, WECK SNG EDGE REORDER POINT 6 REORDER QTY 4
LOC. 24 M-0240 CS/50 NURSES CAPS, GREEN REORDER POINT 3 REORDER QTY 2		LOC. 24 M-0250 CS/50 CATHETERS, OXYGEN, K-20 DISPOSABLE 14FR REORDER POINT 6 REORDER QTY 3

Table 10-12 Vendor Performance Report

DATE 040580

VENDOR PERFORMANCE REPORT   PERIOD 010180 - 033180

P.O. NR.	CODE NR	ITEM DESCRIPTION	UNIT ORDERED	QTY	UNIT COST	ORDER DATE	DATE TO RECEIVE	DATE RECEIVED	QUANTITY RECEIVED	MESSAGE
01938		SMITH STATIONARY SUPPLY COMPANY								
50100	AE010	ENVELOPES, WHITE 9 1/2 X 4	BX/500	8	4.18	010980	012380	021480*	8	LATE
	AF080	BACTERIOLOGY STRIPS LIGHT BLUE BORDER	PG/100	10	3.99	010980	012380	012380	10	
50310	AF200	RADIOLOGIC REPORT	PG/500	6	9.50	012080	013080	012680	6	
50315	AF155	NAME CARDS	PG/1000	10	4.95	012180	020380	020380* 021080*	5 5	PARTIAL PARTIAL

TOTAL LINE ITEMS ORDERED   4
TOTAL LINE ITEMS COMPLETED 1ST SHIPMENT   3
PERCENT COMPLETED 1ST SHIPMENT   .75

Table 10-13 Nonissued Item Report

DATE 010380

NON ISSUED ITEM REPORT

CODE	ITEM DESCRIPTION	UNIT	UNIT COST	QTY O/H	TOTAL COST	LAST ISSUE DATE
MC125	CRUTCH TIPS	PR	2.10	8	16.80	110579
ME007	ELECTRODES, DISP #2241	BG/25	9.00	3	27.00	072479
MM130	MEDICINE CUPS, 1 OZ	TU/100	0.50	12	6.00	091579
				TOTAL	49.80	

Conversion to the Computer

The conversion process requires a number of important steps that must be taken by many people to produce a successful system. Conversion is a team effort requiring the involvement of data processing, accounting, purchasing, and the inventory practitioner. Because of the coordination involved, the individual with the ultimate responsibility for the inventory (materiel manager or inventory practitioner) should retain primary responsibility for the conversion.

The major phases of a conversion to the computer are:

1. cost analysis, preliminary system design, and administrative approval
2. detailed system design, testing of programs, procedures, and debugging
3. preparation for conversion
4. system testing
5. conversion or system upload
6. followup

For hospitals that do not already have an in-house computer, it may be necessary to include a phase for equipment selection. This phase would be inserted between phases 1 and 2.

As has been noted in this section, system design is the foundation of any computerization effort. Simply introducing a computerized inventory control system that has not been soundly developed cannot make it an outstanding system. Design of a system is the most difficult phase, and its importance cannot be overemphasized.

Two avenues of approach are available to the practitioner in the development of an inventory software package. The first is obtaining a general software package from a computer manufacturer. These software packages can be acquired for $1500 to $2500 per month, including the necessary hardware. These general software packages can be modified by hospital data processing personnel or the manufacturer to meet the hospital's requirements.

The second alternative is for the hospital to develop its own software. This alternative will entail many hours of time by the practitioner and data processing personnel. Programs must be written, tested, and debugged. Every facet of the system will require a significant amount of attention to detail and planning. But although developing your own software may appear to be an impossible task, it is not.

Whether a software package is purchased or developed in house, responsibility for each phase of the conversion process must be detailed. Data must be collected and verified for accuracy and completeness. Special forms may have to be designed, people trained, and procedures rewritten. The attention to detail is a paramount necessity. For this reason, the use of a PERT (program evaluation review technique) chart will prove to be invaluable. Prior to the actual conversion, a detailed systems test should be conducted that includes the following:

1. All clerical procedures should be tested. The actual flow of documentation and quality control procedures should be checked.
2. The entire computer system should be tested by data processing to ensure that program interface is correct, and that the operators have the necessary information to execute all programs.
3. After the systems test by data processing, a complete parallel test should be conducted. During the parallel test, actual documentation should be processed through the system and verified to the manual system. A group of selected A items should be used for this purpose. The parallel test will provide for some hands-on training for departmental personnel to familiarize them with the new procedures. The parallel operation also will serve to ensure that the system is debugged.
4. Immediately prior to the actual conversion, a complete physical inventory should be conducted and verified for accuracy. All routine purchasing, receiving, and issuing procedures should be suspended until the conversion is completed.

The final phase of the conversion process is the followup, which should last for three to six months after upload. Specifically, the following items should be covered:

• Are the new procedures working? Is anyone having difficulty with forms, reports, etc.?

• Are the objectives being met?

• Is the system doing everything it was designed to accomplish?

• Are the users satisfied with the system?

USE OF QUANTITATIVE METHODS

Regardless of whether a hospital uses a manual or computerized perpetual inventory system, three basic questions must be addressed. Because inventory practitioners are most often working with limited resources, it is important to determine the items or groups of items that deserve a maximum control effort. The classification of inventory items into groups by annual dollar value of usage is called ABC analysis. As a quantitative method, ABC analysis answers the first question of *what* items deserve the greatest amount of control.

The second, and most critical, question to be answered is *when* an item is to be ordered. The determination of when an order is to be generated forms the basis for establishing safety stock that will have a direct relationship to levels of service provided to the various hospital departments.

The final question to be addressed is that of *how much* to order when an order is placed. Practitioners often struggle with this question in an effort to achieve an economical balance between cost to order and cost of possession. The two most accepted methods used to answer the questions of how much and when to order are order point/economic order quantity and the periodic ordering system.

ABC ANALYSIS

ABC analysis is a quantitative technique used to focus attention on and apply effort to items that will yield the greatest results. Developed by Vilfredo Pareto, an Italian economist, ABC analysis has also been referred to as "Pareto's law." Simply stated, ABC analysis assumes that 10 percent of the inventory line items provide 70 percent of the total annual dollar value of issues. These are "A" items. The next 20 percent of the inventory line items provide 20 percent of the total annual dollar value of issues. These are "B" items. Finally, the remaining 70 percent of the inventory line items provide 10 percent of the total annual dollar value of issues. These are the "C" items. Figure 10-1 presents a graphic illustration of this technique.

As a quantitative technique, ABC analysis tries to isolate the vital few items, A and B, so that the bulk of the inventory practitioner's time can be devoted to controlling these items.

The following steps are necessary in quantifying an ABC analysis.

1. Calculate the annual usage in units for each inventory item.
2. Multiply the annual usage in units by the latest unit cost to arrive at the annual usage in dollars for each item.
3. Rank the items from highest total annual dollars to lowest total annual dollars and assign categories based upon the 10-20-70 concept.

One question that often arises is why is there the need to quantify by total annual dollars and not simply by usage in units? The answer is that annual usage, without applying a dollar value, yields no meaningful common factor for making a valid comparison. For example, to give the same amount of control to large paper clips with an annual issue of 1,328 units as to 390 units of open heart custom pump packs may be unwise. The annual dollar value of issues for the large paper clips may amount to only $637, as opposed to $50,000 for the annual value of issues for the open heart custom pump packs. A stock-out of paper clips may cause an incon-

Figure 10-1 Graphic Illustration of ABC Analysis

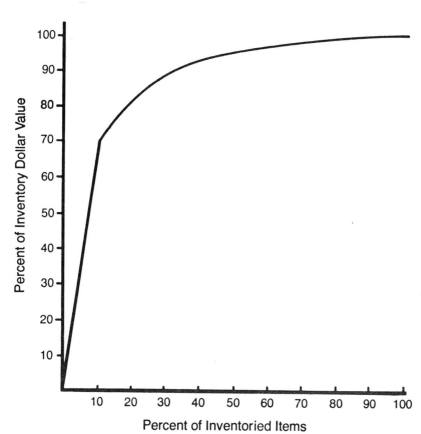

venience for someone, but a stock-out of open heart custom pump packs could endanger a patient's life. See Table 10-14 for an example of ABC analysis.

The time required to quantify the inventory items for an ABC analysis is extensive and will vary according to the size of any given inventory. Any amount of time spent on this type of analysis requires some return on investment. The payoff for the time spent comes in two areas. First, the purchasing practitioner's time can be better spent in negotiating to reduce the unit costs of an A item over a C item. Second, the inventory practitioner can devote more time to controlling A and B items to prevent stock-outs and reduce inventory balances (safety stock, on hand, etc.). Stated another way, the time spent by limited human resources on the use of limited financial resources results in tangible cost effectiveness.

Table 10-14 Example of ABC Analysis

Item Number	Stock Number	Description	Annual Usage	Annual Dollars
1	MO-10	Oxygenators	67 cs	$54,270
2	MP-124	Pump Packs, custom	392 ea	50,568
3	MS-60	Sponge, Lap., 18×18	632 cs	32,548
4	MP-105	Probe Covers	454 bx	17,620
5	MU-40	Underpads	462 cs	14,438
6	MN-38	Needle, 20g×1¼'' #2878	235 bx	14,100
7	MC-133	Cardiotomy Reservoir	420 ea	13,440
8	MP-31	Pad, Back, Grounding	154 cs	12,782
9	MF-05	Filter, arterial blood	66 cs	12,672
10	MF-06	Filter, cardiotomy	65 cs	12,090
		ETC.		
46	MT-40	Tube, endotracheal, #8	1760 ea	3,644
		Total All A Items		$489,941

The results of an ABC analysis should also be used to establish separate inventory control policies for each classification. These policies should govern the following areas:

- forecasting techniques

- order quantity determination

- safety stock calculation

- lead time determination

- issuance of stock to using departments

- perpetual inventory records versus physical control

Forecasting techniques for A and B items, of necessity, require a more diligent effort than for C items. This effort can be implemented through improved communication between the inventory practitioner and the using departments.

One method of improved communication can be accomplished during the hospital budgeting process. Typically, the budgeting process requires department managers to forecast patient census, number and type of operations, number of laboratory procedures, and x-ray examinations. This type of information, properly communicated to the inventory practitioner, can provide the necessary coordination between forecasted patient load changes and the supplies necessary to support these changes. Anticipated changes in the medical staff is also important information for the practitioner because of the impact on supply usage.

Improved communication between the user and the practitioner can have a tremendous impact on the cost effectiveness of inventory management. In a majority of cases, it will be incumbent upon the practitioner to initiate the communication process. Why the practitioner? Experience has shown that most department managers are concerned with personnel and capital budget requirements, with only a cursory look at supply requirements. Most often, this cursory look results in merely adding a percentage figure for inflation and changes in procedures for each departmental budget. Little, if any, effort is made to coordinate the departmental supply budgets with the inventory budget. This lack of coordination can result in either overstatements or understatements of anticipated supply costs for both the user departments and the inventory.

To resolve the problem, the practitioner should work with the finance department to improve the budget process. Typical changes may include: (1) separating the dollars budgeted for supplies into two categories, inventory supplies and direct purchase supplies; and (2) requiring department managers to forecast anticipated need for high usage A and B items. This information, analyzed and coordinated by the practitioner, can be invaluable. Comparisons between forecasted departmental needs and actual history can lead to realistic and more accurate budgeting for the departments and improved supply forecasting by the practitioner.

Not only will this coordination process aid the inventory practitioner, but it also can provide assistance to the purchasing department for competitive bidding and negotiation. Communication through information sharing can lead to improved forecasting and inventory control techniques required for good inventory management.

The second policy area, order quantity determination, will lead to the decision as to which quantitative technique can be best applied to each inventory item or classification. Later in this chapter, the use of order point/economic order quantity and the periodic order system will be explained in greater detail to enable the practitioner to determine which system is best suited to answer the order quantity question.

Because ABC analysis allows for selective inventory control, safety stocks for A and B items should be kept low, since these items are to be subjected to close scrutiny. C items, which are not subject to the same tight control, afford the possibility for higher safety stocks to prevent large numbers of stock-outs.

ABC analysis also lends itself to closer coordination of normal lead times from the vendor. Because of their annual dollar value, A and B items should be closely coordinated between the inventory and the vendor. Vendor stocking of A and B items is critical to lower inventories and safety stock. The track record of vendor deliveries becomes critical in the determination of lead time demand.

The method and quantities issued to using departments of A and B items also should be reviewed by the practitioner. Selective controls should not end once an item is issued from inventory. Items that are high dollar value to the storeroom are high dollar value items to the using departments. Quantitative control should also be extended to unofficial inventory in user departments. Remember, inventory management extends beyond the walls of the storeroom. Time expended in analyzing and quantifying user usage can and will provide an important aid in forecasting and management of the hospital's supply dollars.

Finally, some thought must be given to whether an item or group of items will be controlled by a perpetual inventory or by a simple physical control method. This decision must be based upon reliance on a perpetual inventory system versus the dollars required to have someone physically check stock on a weekly or other basis.

By now the value of ABC analysis should be clear. The ABC principle is universal. It is a basic principle that should be applied in any inventory management program. The professional inventory practitioner who understands the ABC principle will be using this principle in many areas of inventory control.

WHEN AND HOW MUCH?

The questions of when to order and how much to order are of critical concern in every inventory management system. Conceptually, two systems have evolved to resolve these questions: order point/economic order quantity and the periodic ordering system. Both of these systems offer unique approaches to inventory management. Because of their uniqueness and the complexities involved, each system will be discussed separately.

ORDER POINT/ECONOMIC ORDER QUANTITY

The combination of order point/economic order quantity is the most widely recognized system for inventory management. The order point portion answers the question of when to order. Economic order quantity answers the question of how much.

Order point is a predetermined quantity that indicates to the inventory practitioner that the potential need for an order has been reached.

Order point is normally expressed in dispensing units. When any given issue of stock causes the balance (on hand plus on order) to drop below this predetermined point, the item requires review.

The order point is usually set at a figure that will satisfy the expected demand between the time the order is placed and when the order is received, otherwise known as lead time. Thus,

Order point = Anticipated lead time issues

Two calculations are required to determine the order point for any given time. The first is the determination of the time (in days) from the day the order is placed until item is received. Whenever possible, the average lead time should be calculated by using a minimum of the last five order periods to determine the average time involved. Close attention should be given to the longest lead time involved. The average should be determined from the raw numbers used and then subtracted from the longest period. The difference between the average and the longest period should be divided in half and added to the average to determine a more accurate reflection of true lead time. Table 10-15 illustrates this calculation method.

A common mistake in determining lead time is to ignore the time between when the requisition is generated and actual order placement. Normally, practitioners tend to consider only the time between order placement by purchasing and its receipt. The primary reason for this mistake is that an assumption is made that the order will be placed by purchasing on the same day the requisition is received. Often this is not the case. Consolidation of orders, minimum dollar requirements for quantity discounts, or grouping items to eliminate paying freight costs all contribute to delaying the order in purchasing. These potentials must be recognized by the inventory practitioner as a legitimate part of the lead time determination. Therefore, lead time should be calculated from the day the requisition is sent to purchasing to the time of receipt.

Table 10-15 Calculating Lead Time

Order Number	Lead Time in Days
1	5
2	8
3	4
4	5
5	7
5		28
	5.8 or 6 days
Longest	8 days
Average	−6 days
Difference	2 days ÷ ½ = 1 day

Lead Time = 6 days + 1 day or 7 days

The second calculation is to determine the amount issued during the lead time period. This figure traditionally has been calculated by dividing total annual issues by 365 days and multiplying the resulting figure by the average lead time. As an illustration,

$$\frac{\text{Total annual issues}}{365 \text{ days}} = \frac{500 \text{ units}}{365 \text{ days}} = 1.37 \times 7 \text{ days} = 9.59, \text{ or } 10 \text{ units}$$

This traditional methodology assumes that demand is static throughout the year and it does not consider variations in user demand. In reality, variations in user demand occur on an almost daily basis.

A more accurate method for determining lead time demand is to use the actual issues that occurred during the same reorder periods used in the calculation for lead time. The same mathematical computation used to determine lead time in days can be applied to this calculation. Table 10-16 illustrates this method of calculation. As you will note, only the highest quantity issued is given additional consideration because of the impact it makes on available stock and the increased possibility of a stock-out.

Table 10-16 Order Point Quantity

Order Number	Lead Time in Days	Quantity Issued
1	5	6
2	8	8
3	4	2
4	5	6
5	7	10

5 ⌊32 Total Issues

6.4 average lead time demand

Highest Amount of Issues	10
Average Amount of Issues	−6.4
Difference	½ ⌊3.6
	1.8

1.8 + 6.4 = 8.2 or 8 units order point quantity

Safety Stock

Despite efforts to calculate the proper order point for any given item, the potential for a stock-out still exists. Vendor back orders and increased demand are still likely to occur. To protect against the possibility of a stock-out, the concept of safety stock has been developed to provide additional protection.

The safety stock portion of the inventory is that amount of stock that is added to the reorder point to meet the need for additional protection against a stock-out. The amount of necessary safety stock is based not on ordering/carrying costs, but on the amount needed for protection against stock outages for each item under consideration. Critical items may require greater protection than less critical items. Each item must be considered separately on the basis of criticalness, accuracy of forecasted usage, actual usage, lead time, average lead time demand, and availability of other vendors to provide the item. With this type of analysis, every effort should be made to avoid using nontypical, nonrecurring situations. Consideration must also be given to the method of computing lead time and lead time demand. If average computations are used, safety stock requirements may be much greater than if the calculation method proposed in this section is used. The suggested method of order point calculations provides consideration for the exception of usage and lead time. Thus, lower safety stocks may be employed.

Where lengthy analysis is not practical, the use of an established standard should be considered. Such a standard can be expressed in days of supply and applied to every inventory item. The exact amount of the standard safety stock is subjective in this instance rather than objective.

Other authors have offered objective approaches to quantifying safety stock requirements in terms of applying probability theorems to lead time demand. These quantitative applications are good techniques and should be considered as an alternative to the across-the-board technique.[1]

Whatever methodology is utilized, it is important to recognize that the use of safety stock will impact the determination of the order point. The formula of order point now becomes:

Order point = Anticipated lead time issues plus safety stock

Economic Order Quantity

Associated with order point is the use of economic order quantity (EOQ) to answer the second question of how much to order. There has long been a conflict between inventory managers and purchasing practitioners with regard to the question of how much. Conflict arises between a low inventory objective and quantity purchasing to achieve lower unit pricing and cost to order. Economic order quantity is perhaps the most widely recognized method of resolving this conflict.

EOQ is most often expressed as a mathematical equation where

$$EOQ = \sqrt{\frac{2 \text{ (Annual usage in units) (Cost to order)}}{\text{(Unit cost) (Inventory carrying costs)}}}$$

For a graphic representation of EOQ, see Figure 10-2.

The use of EOQ should result in achieving the lowest total cost for procurement and the cost of carrying inventory.

Despite the almost universal acceptance of the EOQ equation, practitioners usually guess or estimate two critical portions of the equation: cost to order and inventory carrying costs. The reason why these two factors are estimated can probably be attributed to either lack of knowledge of how to perform the calculation or lack of time. The former can be dealt with here; the latter cannot.

Cost to order is calculated by dividing the total cost associated with the purchasing cycle by the number of purchase orders written in a given year. The figures required include:

Figure 10-2 Graphic Illustration of EOQ

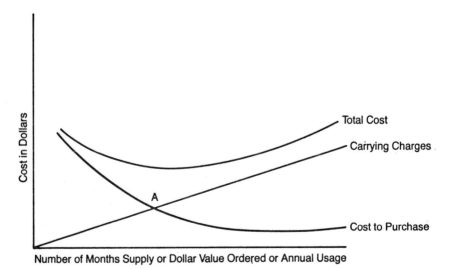

EOQ occurs at point A, which is the point of lowest total cost for purchasing and inventory carrying costs.

, salaries (purchasing, accounts payable, and receiving)

• taxes paid (FICA)

, benefits

• depreciation associated with each of the above departments

• apportioned insurance costs

• apportioned costs for utilities

• supply costs

While most practitioners do not have all of these figures at their fingertips, the necessary information is usually available from hospital financial departments. Why include the costs of accounts payable and receiving? The most fundamental reason is that you are seeking a total cost figure. The costs associated with receiving the merchandise and paying the invoice are legitimate costs in the purchasing cycle and should not be ignored.

Once the total costs have been identified, two additional pieces of information are needed to complete the calculation: the number of purchase orders written for a year and the number of line items ordered. Total line items are divided by total purchase orders to determine the average line items per order. For example, a hospital that writes 7,620 purchase orders per year for 20,760 line items would have 2.7 average line items per order.

Once the average line items per order are established, the total annual costs are divided by the total purchase orders written. The resulting figure is the average cost per purchase order. To illustrate this point, let us assume that total annual costs amount to $80,000. When divided by total purchase orders written (7,620), the average cost per purchase order is $10.49.

The final step is to divide the average cost to order by the average line items per order, or

$$\frac{\$10.49}{2.7} = \$3.88$$

It is the average cost per line item that is used for the calculation of EOQ.

Why use cost to order by line item and not the cost of a purchase order? The answer lies in the fact that, normally, multiple items are placed on a purchase order. Assuming this to be true, EOQ seeks the cost to place one order for that single item. Unless the average lines per purchase order are less than 1.5, the cost of an average purchase order will distort the EOQ formula unnecessarily. Any hospital with an average of 1.5 lines per purchase order should examine its procedures because it is unnecessarily increasing the total cost of placing an order. It is also important to remember that the purpose of EOQ is to achieve a balance between cost to order and inventory carrying costs.

Inventory carrying costs are determined much the same as cost to order. The following figures are necessary for this calculation:

- salaries (storeroom personnel)

- taxes paid (FICA)

- benefits

- depreciation

- insurance costs (building and inventory)

- apportioned cost of utilities

- routine supply costs

- cost of obsolescence and shrinkage

- alternative investment costs

Each of these figures is expressed as a percentage of the ending inventory dollar value; that is, the individual total cost divided by the total dollar value of ending inventory. When the percentages are added together, they will equal the true inventory carrying costs for the inventory.

Experienced practitioners may wonder if it is really necessary to go through the time and effort required for these two calculations. Why not simply use a figure of $15 per order and 25 to 30 percent inventory carrying costs? To these practitioners the answer is that either figure overstated in the EOQ equation can result in some significant variances in the average inventory. As you will note, Table 10-17 is an example of overstating both cost to order and inventory carrying costs. The result of the overstatement of costs is an overstock of 106 units tying up $530 in additional capital.

Obviously, this problem has been simplified for use as an example to make a point—any figure used that is not accurate can lead to costly overstocks for the hospital. The reader should recognize that the severity of impact for any given hospital will depend upon the extent of the overstatement of costs when compared with the actual figures. Remember too, the example cited is for only one item. This situation, applied to any given total inventory, could result in hundreds or thousands of dollars tied up in inventory overstocks.

Practitioners should also be aware that variances in the EOQ equation will also affect the inventory turnover rate. The greater the overstock, the lower the turnover

Table 10-17 Overstatement of Costs

	Problem A	Problem B
Annual Usage in Units	1,000	1,000
Cost to Order	$30.00	$3.00
Unit Cost	$ 5.00	$5.00
Inventory Carrying Cost	45%	37%
Safety Stock in Units	15	15
Substituting:		
1	$\sqrt{\dfrac{2(1000)(30)}{5(.45)}}$	$\sqrt{\dfrac{2(1000)(3)}{5(.37)}}$
2	$\sqrt{\dfrac{60,000}{2.25}}$	$\sqrt{\dfrac{46,000}{1.85}}$
3	$\sqrt{26,666.66}$	$\sqrt{3,243.24}$
4.	163.30	56.9
	or 163	57

Average Inventory = Safety Stock + ½ Order Quantity

Problem A   15 + 163 = 178 × $5.00 = $890.00

Problem B   15 + 57 = 72 × $5.00 = $360.00

Overstock   106 $530.00

rate. Later in this chapter the question of inventory turnover rate is explored in greater detail.

The question as to when these calculations should be made is important and requires an answer. The end of the fiscal year appears to be the optimum time for this procedure. Normally, budgets have been completed and anticipated salary increases and other expenses have been projected for the forthcoming fiscal year. Most annual inventories are taken at the end of the fiscal year, and the required information is also available for an ABC analysis. Thus, the end of the fiscal year (or early in the first quarter of the new year) is an excellent time to determine costs for the coming or new fiscal year. Practitioners are also advised to review inventory carrying costs if there are radical changes in the prime interest rate and/or during periods of double digit inflation. Changes in the prime interest rate and inflation can have a severe impact on inventory carrying costs. In addition, practitioners should consider reviewing A and B items at the midpoint of the fiscal year on the basis of changes in forecasted demand for usage, patient census, and patient mix. Fluctuations in any of these variables will have a definite effect on the inventory. With 70 percent of annual dollars invested in these items, they require a maximum amount of control.

As a quantitative technique, EOQ fixes the order quantity and the timing of order placement becomes variable, depending upon actual demand. The fixed order quantity of EOQ has been criticized for having two basic shortcomings. The first is that EOQ assumes a fixed purchase price of each item and offers little consideration for quantity discounts. For this reason, it has been suggested that the total annual unit costs be calculated using discount prices and then compared with the standard methodology. The EOQ used by the hospital should be the one that yields the lowest total annual costs. As a practical matter, this criticism appears to be in error, since the practitioner should be dealing with committed annual volume when negotiating or bidding unit pricing. Commitment of annual volume should be sufficient to yield pricing equal to the quantity discounts offered. It is important to recognize that vendors who offer quantity discounts do so to combat the actions of purchasing practitioners who tend to wander aimlessly from vendor to vendor. Purchasing practitioners are responsible for obtaining the best pricing available. Inventory practitioners are responsible for maintaining low inventories with high turnover, and must use the pricing obtained by purchasing for the calculation of EOQ. Lower total annual cost is the primary reason for using EOQ, and to that end it goes beyond simple unit pricing to encompass purchasing and inventory carrying costs. Thus, the criticism that EOQ does not consider quantity discounts is certainly on shaky ground.

The second criticism is that EOQ does not take case quantity into consideration for items issued in less than full case units of measure. This criticism is well founded, but in response, the consideration of the use of common sense is offered. It is obvious that when EOQ results in an order quantity of 95 each for an item that is packed 100 per case, the EOQ is adjusted to meet the case quantity! For items where the calculated EOQ is significantly less than the case quantity (i.e., EOQ = 60, case quantity = 100), consideration should be given to purchasing the item from another hospital. Similar consideration should be given to finding out if this item is really needed. Experience has shown that this situation occurs primarily with low volume C items.

EOQ is a sound inventory management technique that will achieve the objective of the inventory and the purchasing practitioner's lower total annual costs.

PERIODIC ORDERING SYSTEM

The periodic ordering system (POS) is the second method by which the inventory manager can answer the question of when and how much to order. Unlike the previously described order point system where the time interval is variable, POS fixes the interval between orders. Purchasing practitioners encourage the use of POS because fixed time periods can be established to coincide with the vendor representative's routine visits. To illustrate this procedure, a particular vendor visits the hospital every two weeks. The review period for that vendor's products could be established to coincide with the visit.

Concise coordination of the vendor visit is not always necessary in order to utilize POS successfully. For example, one practitioner who utilized POS placed large orders at the beginning of the month for routine inventory items. Nonroutine orders were placed weekly to coincide with the vendor's visit. When queried about this ordering pattern, the practitioner responded that the vendor's terms were net 30 days, which meant the hospital processed the vendor's check on the tenth of the month following delivery. By placing a large order at the beginning of the month, combined with the vendor's reliable delivery of two or three days, the practitioner was using the vendor's money for the time period between receipt of merchandise and payment of the invoice. The net result was stock on hand and available for issue without tying up the hospital's financial resources.

Use of POS is advantageous for the purchasing practitioner, but how does it work for the inventory practitioner? It has already been noted that POS answers the question of when to order by fixing the time interval between order periods. How does POS answer the question of how much? Unlike EOQ, where the order quantity is fixed and the time interval is variable, POS fixes the interval and the order quantity becomes the variable. Thus, the order quantity for any given item depends upon usage during the fixed time interval. Orders are placed for the quantity necessary to bring on-hand stocks up to a desired maximum level.

The use of POS as an inventory management tool is practical when one or more of the following situations exist:

- The item(s) warrants tight control because of high usage and frequent orders.
- A perpetual inventory control system is not utilized.
- Consolidation of the number of items ordered from a given vendor will reduce unit pricing, transportation, or purchasing costs.
- Issuance of the item(s) is at irregular intervals.
- Excessively long delivery periods exist.

While POS is easily applied to a hospital inventory, it does have a number of disadvantages. First, while the review period may be determined for convenience, such periods should also take into consideration the annual value of the item versus the cost of the review. High dollar volume items should be reviewed on a more frequent basis when the review costs can be offset by reducing the average cost of inventory and the inventory carrying costs.

Second, POS does not lessen or eliminate the need for adequate safety stock. Because of unanticipated fluctuations in usage and possible delivery failure by the vendor, safety stocks may provide either too little or too much protection for any specific item. Therefore, care must be exercised in setting safety stocks.

Third, because POS does not specifically define either a predetermined order point quantity or order quantity, reordering tends to become automatic, which, if not carefully controlled, can lead to an overstock situation.

Finally, the establishment of a desired maximum level usually requires the inventory practitioner to experiment on a trial-and-error basis to achieve a balance between order costs and inventory carrying costs. Normally, a compromise has to be reached. Purchasing practitioners have long held the position that ordering more frequently than once per month per item will usually result in higher purchasing costs. Inventory managers have also stated that ordering large quantities may lead to excessive overstocks with higher inventory carrying costs. Taken together, all of the aforementioned disadvantages can lead the inventory practitioner into a dense cloud bank with little, if any, sense of direction of how to apply POS. So let us clear the air about how to use a periodic ordering system.

As previously mentioned, the critical determination in using POS is the establishment of a review period—and this often means a conflict between the purchasing and inventory practitioners. This conflict can be resolved using a quantitative method that balances cost to order and inventory carrying costs. The formula is similar to EOQ, and simply stated is

$$P = \sqrt{\frac{I}{2}\frac{A}{C}}$$

where

P = number of orders per year
I = inventory carrying costs expressed as a percent
A = annual requirements in dollars (annual units × price)
C = ordering costs per line item in dollars

As with EOQ, determining inventory carrying costs and cost per order is critical to determining the number of orders per year. The same calculation methods should be used as developed for EOQ.

The following illustration will assist in understanding the calculation method for establishing a review period.

A = 1000 units × $5/unit = $5000
I = 37 percent
C = $3

Substituting in the formula,

$$P = \sqrt{\frac{I}{2} \quad \frac{A}{C}}$$

$$P = \sqrt{\frac{(0.37)}{(2)} \quad \frac{(5000)}{(3)}}$$

$$P = \sqrt{\frac{1850}{6}}$$

$$P = \sqrt{308.34}$$

$$P = 17.56, \text{ or 18 orders per year}$$

Once the number of review periods (orders) per year is known, the next step is to convert this number into periods of days or weeks. This is done by dividing weeks (or days) in a year by P. Simply stated, the review period *(RP)* equals

$$RP = \frac{52}{P}$$

Using our example, the review period will occur every three weeks or 20 days.

$$\text{Weeks: } RP = \frac{52}{18} = 2.88 \text{ weeks}$$

$$\text{Days: } RP = \frac{365}{18} = 20.2 \text{ days}$$

Now that the review period has been determined, the next step is to determine safety stock. Under POS, safety stock becomes a subjective decision. That is, the inventory practitioner establishes a standard for the desired amount of protection to be afforded to each item. For example, the necessary safety stock for an A item may be judged to be five days' protection. Using information from our previous example, the safety stock for the item would be 14 units.

$$\frac{1000}{365} \times 5 \text{ days} = 13.69, \text{ or 14 units}$$

With the establishment of safety stock, the desired maximum can be calculated. The desired maximum is equal to the average usage during the review period plus safety stock. Using our previous example, it has been established that the annual usage equals 1,000 units, safety stock equals 14 units, and the review period is every 21 days. Therefore,

$$\text{Desired maximum} = \frac{1000 \text{ units}}{365 \text{ days}} \times 21 \text{ days} + 14 \text{ units, or 22 units}$$

All of the calculations for POS are now complete with the exception of order quantity. Earlier it was established that the order quantity is the variable when using POS. When the review period occurs, the order quantity is determined by subtracting the actual on-hand balance from the desired maximum and adding anticipated lead time demand usage. To illustrate this procedure, assume a desired maximum of 25 units, an on-hand balance of 15 units, delivery time of five days, and lead time usage of five units. The order quantity becomes

Desired maximum	25 units
On-hand balance	−15 units
Lead time usage	+ 5 units
Order quantity	15 units

Many inventory practitioners who use POS fail to recognize the need to calculate an order quantity that includes anticipated lead time usage. This oversight is the single greatest mistake made when POS is used. Failure to anticipate lead time usage will increase the possibility of a stock-out by a substantial margin.

ORDER POINT VERSUS PERIODIC CONTROL

The question of which system is better always comes up in conversations involving inventory management. Among inventory practitioners, order point is the simplest to apply, and the most popular. Yet, in hospitals where departmental inventories are not under the control of one central manager, periodic ordering is the system most often utilized.

From a practical perspective, a combination of these two systems appears to work well. Of course, it depends upon how large a hospital is involved and how much control is exerted over other departmental inventories.

In central stores, POS is excellent for use on forms, office supplies, x-ray film, IV solutions, and other commodities purchased from one vendor under system contracts. POS is also the basis for control of exchange cart and PAR level programs.

Order point is more practical for nonsystem control items in central stores. The right system for use in any hospital is a matter of judgment as to which system will provide the necessary control and meet the goals of the hospital.

STOCK ROTATION

Spoilage is a problem that the inventory practitioner must deal with on a daily basis. A good stock rotation program can help to reduce the spoilage problem. Broadly speaking, spoilage occurs when an item is no longer fit for its intended use. While physical damage to the container or package certainly applies to spoilage, the age of an item is most often the primary problem for inventory items.

The introduction of sterile disposable products seemed to heighten the awareness of a product's useful shelf life. Shelf life refers to a specific time period, designated by the manufacturer, within which a product is considered to be usable. The shelf life can be as short as 30 days or as long as five years, depending upon the conditions under which the item is stored. Although most practitioners equate shelf life only with items having an expiration date, it should be recognized that every item has a limited life cycle. If unused over a long period of time, every item, regardless of composition, will begin to break down and lose some of its original properties. For example, paper packaging used for catheters will begin to yellow if left on a shelf unused for two years or more.

Stock rotation does not have to be complicated. Two simple procedures are all that is required. First, clearly mark the month and year on the external carton when the item is received. And second, place new merchandise either behind or under the oldest merchandise. Both of these practices take only a few minutes and will help to reduce losses from spoilage.

INVENTORY PERFORMANCE INDICATORS

The final element in a sound inventory management program is the measurement of the program's success. Quantitatively, turnover rate, dollars per bed, and days of inventory are the most acceptable measurement methods available.

Turnover Rate

Inventory turnover is the quantitative measurement of the number of times that total inventory dollars are issued and replaced. The turnover rate is calculated by dividing the total annual dollars for supplies issued by the dollar value of the ending inventory. For example, if the dollar value of annual issues is $760,000 and the ending inventory dollar value is $88,500, then the turnover rate is equal to:

$$\frac{\$760,000}{\$\ 88,500} = 8.58$$

The question most often asked by practitioners is: What constitutes a good inventory turnover rate? Many experts feel that an acceptable minimum turnover rate for any inventory is 12 times per year. However, many practitioners in the field, including this author, believe eight to ten turns per year to be realistic. Conversely, a turnover rate of six or less is inadequate and requires some type of additional analysis and corrective action. Practitioners should also recognize that the hospital's proximity to suppliers and the bed density of the area will influence the determination of an acceptable turnover rate. For example, a rural community hospital in western Nebraska may not be capable of, or want to achieve, a turnover rate of 10 or 12. On the other hand, a hospital located in a major metropolitan area such as New York or Chicago may, and probably should, achieve a turnover rate in excess of 12 to 18 turns.

What do you do in cases where the absolute size of the inventory continues to grow? An increase in the absolute size of the inventory is not meaningful until it is related to issues. Inventories grow through the addition of new items, increased demand for items already in inventory, and reduced demand for items that have not been properly identified.

The next question is almost academic: How can inventory turnover be improved? The way to get a faster turnover rate is, first, to clean out surplus and reduce slow-moving items. The second way is to concentrate on increasing the turnover on A items. The third method is to reduce the amount of safety stock and the lead time required to order and receive replacement stocks. Practitioners should be aware that reduction in safety stock will increase the probability of a stock-out. If this method is chosen, it should be used selectively.

Dollars per Bed

The quantitative method for determining inventory dollars per bed is to divide the ending inventory dollar figure by the average number of occupied beds during the year. Notice that the methodology specifies occupied beds, not total beds. Occupied beds provide a more accurate picture of the inventory activity and need for inventory. For example, as Table 10-18 shows, inventory dollars per bed when calculated using total beds reflect $220 per bed, which, by some standards, would indicate a "good" amount of control. However, when the calculation is made on the basis of average occupancy, the dollars per bed increase to $293.33, which, again by some standards, would be indicative of "poor" inventory control and probably of excessive inventory.

The question is, when does an inventory practitioner begin to recognize that inventory dollars per bed are too high? The answer goes beyond the traditional beliefs of compensating for poor vendor performance, and a lack of effective systems, and depends upon a number of additional factors; these include the type of hospital, length of stay, types of items maintained within the inventory,

Table 10-18 Inventory Dollars per Bed

Hospital Size. 400 beds

Medical/Surgical Inventory Value: $88,000.00

Percent of Occupancy: 75% or 300 Beds

A. Calculation by Total Beds

$$\frac{\$88,000}{400 \text{ Beds}} = \$220.00 \text{ per Bed}$$

B. Calculation by Average Occupancy

$$\frac{\$88,000}{300 \text{ Beds}} = \$293.33 \text{ per Bed}$$

inventory turnover rates, changes in medical staff, poor forecasting, rate of inflation, and types of patients treated. This last factor has, perhaps, the greatest impact. Types of patients treated means the general patient population; that is, medical patients versus surgical patients. Although patient mix may not have a great impact on a large hospital (400-plus beds), it definitely does have an effect in the smaller hospital.

It is obvious that the greater the percentage of surgical patients, the greater the demand for medical/surgical supplies. If a hospital experiences a drop in the surgical patient population, the demand for supplies also drops. Unfortunately, this type of information is not normally communicated to the inventory practitioner and excessive inventory begins to accumulate. Inventory practitioners should recognize that it is not unrealistic to find A items becoming C items in a matter of weeks. Conversely, C items can become A items practically overnight. Thus, it is incumbent upon the inventory practitioner to evaluate all of the factors that can contribute to excessive inventory.

As to judging the performance of any inventory management program on the basis of dollars per bed, practitioners must continually strive toward a reduction in this area. Value judgments of good, fair, and poor performance cannot be made by outside sources; they must be made by the practitioners. Goal setting is important in any inventory reduction program. Practitioners should set realistic goals concerning inventory dollars per bed, while remembering the ultimate objective: to have the right supplies, at the right time, at the lowest cost.

Days of Inventory

Days of inventory refer to the average number of days that an inventory will last without resupply. This measurement is made by dividing the ending inventory dollar value by the average dollar value of issues per day. For example, using an ending inventory value of $88,000, total annual issues of $741,000, and a 365-day year, the days of inventory equal 43.35:

$$\left(\frac{\$\,88,000}{\frac{\$741,000}{365}} \right) = \frac{\$\,88,000}{\$2030.14} = 43.35 \text{ days of inventory}$$

This method has been questioned as to its relevance as a performance indicator, and its use has been limited. It is presented here only as another quantitative measurement relating to inventory performance.

ANNUAL INVENTORY

As a general practice, hospitals are required to "take" a physical count of all items within the official inventory on an annual basis. This physical count is used to verify the available inventory assets at the end of the fiscal year versus accounting's book inventory. The term "book inventory" refers to the inventory dollars that accounting maintains on the official financial records.

Many inventory practitioners and storeroom personnel view this counting procedure as the least attractive part of their jobs, describing it as boring, uninteresting, and a waste of time "because nobody cares anyway." But aside from these general opinions, the annual inventory is one of the most important activities to be performed.

Annual physical inventories force the inventory practitioner to look at the actual activity of every inventory item, review for item duplication, identify shrinkage and obsolescence, and reconcile physical counts with balances posted to the perpetual inventory system.

Preparation

Preparation for the annual inventory should begin several weeks prior to the actual count. Central stores personnel should make sure that items are in their proper locations and that stock is unpacked and stored properly. Inventory sheets should be typed, and should list stock number, description, and unit of measure. These should be prepared from the stores catalog. If the hospital has a computerized inventory, a request should be sent to data processing for an inventory master listing and count sheets.

One week prior to the physical count, all requests for stock and receiving reports should be annotated with the words "Before Inventory." This procedure will identify postings for inventory control and accounts payable.

If the inventory manager intends to terminate routine activities of issue and receipt, a letter should be sent to all departments and vendors informing them when stores will be closed. Hospital departments should also be informed of the proper procedure for obtaining "emergency" supplies from stores during the inventory period. As a matter of routine, all requests for supplies during the counting period require the approval of the inventory practitioner before supplies are released.

One or two days prior to the physical counting, all involved personnel should review the procedures to be used. This gives everyone an opportunity to ask questions and to resolve unforeseen problems.

Actual Count

Before the actual counting begins, stores personnel should be assigned specific areas of responsibility. Actual counting can be accomplished either in teams or by individuals working alone. If the team concept is employed, one person acts as the counter and the other as the recorder. Individuals working alone obviously are responsible for both counting and recording. Regardless of which concept is used, specific areas of the storeroom should be assigned; for example, bulk storage, loose issue, aisles, etc. Some inventory practitioners like to assign specific commodity groups to teams or individuals regardless of where the items are stored. This particular procedure tends to increase the possibility that items might be missed during the counting.

Actual counts should be recorded on individual count sheets, that is, one count sheet per item. Exhibit 10-6 shows a count sheet. This form has two parts. Once the item is counted and recorded on the sheet, both copies are maintained with the stock until the inventory is completed. Each count sheet is prenumbered for control purposes and to ensure that all count sheets are accounted for once the inventory is completed.

During the time the physical count is being taken, the practitioner or someone from accounting should check the completed counts to verify their accuracy. At least 10 percent of all items should be checked. If personnel work overtime, the number of items checked should be increased. This is necessary because the fatigue factor will increase the possibility of errors. To help offset the fatigue factor, all personnel should be required to take breaks (one in the morning and one in the afternoon), lunch, and dinner (if applicable). Such breaks should be mandatory, not an option.

Once the counting and checking have been completed, every area should be double checked to ascertain that every item stored in that area has been counted. Personnel should be assigned to check areas other than the ones they counted. This

Exhibit 10-6 Inventory Count Sheet

```
┌─────────────────────────────────────────────────────────┐
│                 ST. FRANCIS HOSPITAL                      │
│                 BLUE ISLAND, ILLINOIS                     │
│                                                           │
│    DATE _____                 │
│    DEPARTMENT _____                 │
│    ITEM NUMBER _____                 │
│    DESCRIPTION _____                 │
│                                                           │
│    _____                │
│    QTY _____ UNIT _____                 │
│    LOCATION _____                 │
│    COUNTED  BY _____                 │
│    CHECKED  BY _____                 │
│    ANNUAL  USAGE _____                 │
│                                                           │
│    21-46                                                  │
└─────────────────────────────────────────────────────────┘
```

is a necessary quality control step to prevent the "I know I counted everything" syndrome.

After completion of the double check, the top copy of every count sheet should be collected. The second copy should remain with the item. All of the count sheets should be arranged in numerical sequence and checked to make sure that every number has been accounted for. The sheets are now ready for posting to the inventory master list.

The individual responsible for posting count sheets to the master list functions as the final step in the quality control process. Stock numbers and item descriptions must be carefully matched. Comparison of quantities and units of measure are of utmost importance as well. One of the most common mistakes that can be made is to post case quantities to units of measure that are "each," and vice versa. When discrepancies are noted, a recheck should be made to determine the correctness of the information.

If a hospital utilizes a manual perpetual inventory, other stores personnel should be assigned to post the perpetual inventory cards with the physical counts from the second copy of the count sheets. Entries on the inventory cards should read something similar to "1980 Physical Inventory."

Store personnel should also be instructed to maintain a listing of differences between the on-hand balance shown on the inventory card and the physical count. This listing should include stock number, a brief description, on-hand quantity shown on the inventory card, and actual physical count, and should be checked to determine why the discrepancy exists. It should also be priced to assist in resolving dollar discrepancies between the actual physical count dollar figure and the accounting department's inventory dollar balance. The resulting figure will also represent the shrinkage that has occurred during the year.

Again, when a manual perpetual inventory is being used, stores personnel should add up all of the issues to determine the annual issues for every item. This information can be obtained either at the time of physical count or as part of the postinventory routine. However it is acquired, the information is necessary for an ABC analysis of the inventory, recalculation of reorder points, EOQs, etc. Following the actual physical count, annual usage is the most important piece of information that is required to improve inventory management.

Postinventory Activity

The time period following the actual physical count is as important as the preparation period. For the first week following the physical inventory, all requisitions and receiving reports should be stamped "After Inventory." This process will lessen the possibility of confusion as to what transaction belongs in what fiscal year. It is important for the inventory practitioner to be aware of the fact that accounting is not only trying to reconcile your inventory, but also to close the books at the end of the fiscal year. The end of the fiscal year is one of the most hectic periods for every accounting department. Therefore, practitioners have a responsibility to provide as much assistance to accounting as possible.

NOTE

1. Dean S. Ammer, *Purchasing and Materials Management for Health Care Institutions* (Lexington, Mass.: D.C. Heath and Company, 1975).

Chapter 11

Inventory Accounting

The need for maintaining inventory brings with it many financial implications. Earlier in this text, discussions centered around the areas of lowering unit costs, safety stocks, and on-hand inventory. We now enter an area that has not been addressed—inventory accounting.

When considering the problems of inventory management, other authors have chosen to ignore inventory accounting. Discussions with many purchasing practitioners have indicated that proper inventory accounting is a source of misunderstanding and confusion. Much of this misunderstanding arises from trying to apply "pure" accounting theory to actual practice without understanding the theory itself. The discussion that follows will address the various methods of inventory accounting, and their impact on inventory systems, patient charge supplies, and proper recordkeeping.

OFFICIAL VERSUS UNOFFICIAL INVENTORY

Hospitals approach inventory accounting differently from manufacturing and retail companies. Manufacturing companies often have different levels of inventory, all of which are official until the product is sold. These various levels include, but are not limited to, raw materials, work in process, and finished goods. Retail companies have one type of inventory—merchandise available for sale. Both manufacturing and retail companies maintain inventory on their books until the product is sold. Inventory in both cases is considered an asset.

When compared with other industries, the approach to inventory accounting by hospitals is both unique and inconsistent—in the sense that both official and unofficial inventories exist throughout the institution.

What is the difference between official and unofficial inventory? To most hospitals, official inventory is the inventory that is maintained in central stores, central supply, dietary, and pharmacy. When inventory is issued or consumed by any of these departments, it is immediately expensed to the department that requested it.

Unofficial inventory is the stock maintained by laboratory, maintenance, nursing units, etc., that is available for use, but is not controlled by any of the official inventory departments. This unofficial inventory includes items requisitioned from official inventory and items purchased directly for use by a department. Everything is expensed upon issue or receipt.

Why expense everything to the departments at time of issue or receipt? The first reason for this practice is that hospitals view inventory not as an asset, but as a liability. The second reason is that hospitals are reimbursed on a cost basis. Therefore, it is in the best interest of the hospital to expense as much as possible, as soon as possible, to ensure reimbursement and to maintain good cash flow.

One of the problems with this practice is that it encourages the investment of a large number of dollars in unofficial inventory that is unnecessary. Again, this is money that could be working for the hospital and represents a primary source of cost containment through the reduction of these unofficial inventories.

Idealistically, hospitals should approach inventory accounting as retail companies do and expense items once they have been consumed either through the treatment of patients or through normal consumption by the department. Hospital financial people will not necessarily agree with this accounting approach, but it certainly is a strong argument for materiel management.

What happens if a hospital converts to accounting for inventory until it is actually consumed? The first result is that the dollars in official inventory increase dramatically. The second thing the conversion does is to permit an accurate accounting of where the hospital's dollars actually are in terms of consumable inventory. Finally, use of this procedure provides a starting point for reducing inventory and gaining a better handle on controlling hospital supply costs.

The best way to begin this accountability procedure is to make it clear when you establish a PAR or exchange cart program that the actual inventory on the carts or in the cabinets belongs to official inventory and will be accounted for as it is used or removed from the cart or cabinet. The implementation of this type of program can set an example of cost reduction that can be accomplished by controlling inventory until it is actually used. This same procedure can be applied to other nonnursing departments as well.

DETERMINING THE COST OF INVENTORY

The method used to determine the cost of inventory usually is chosen by the hospital's controller. Practitioners generally do not have any input into the decision. It is, however, important that the practitioner understand the method that is utilized and the impact that it will have on inventory cost accounting.

Pure accounting theory states that the cost of any inventory is composed of the purchase price and all other costs incurred in the procurement and distribution process. For hospitals, this is not necessarily the case. It is true that these costs exist, but hospitals treat them as overhead expense and they are not directly applied to the inventory itself. For the purposes of this discussion, the cost of inventory will be limited to purchase price.

One of the most significant complications in determining inventory costs arises when identical units of a particular item have been purchased at different per unit costs during the year. When this is the case, it is necessary to determine the unit price to be associated with the items remaining on hand. The following illustration will clarify the exact nature of this problem.

Assume that during the fiscal year four cases of an IV solution were available for issue. One case was in inventory at the beginning of the year.

Date		Units	Cost
1/1/80	Inventory	1	$18.00
2/27/80	Purchase	1	$18.00
5/30/80	Purchase	1	$18.00
9/30/80	Purchase	1	$22.00
	Total	4	$76.00
	Average cost		$19.00

During the fiscal year, three cases of IV solution were issued, leaving an on-hand balance of one case at the end of the fiscal year. The hospital does not utilize an inventory system or cost accounting, and thus, information as to which cases were issued and which remain is not available. This lack of specific information makes it necessary to adopt an arbitrary assumption as to the flow of costs for the items through the inventory. To resolve this cash flow determination, three methods have been developed:

1. cash flow in the order in which the expenditures were made
2. cash flow in the reverse order in which the expenditures were made
3. cash flow as an average of the expenditures for the item

Use of any of these methods will affect the cost of inventory to varying degrees, as you will soon see.

First In, First Out

The first in, first out (FIFO) method is based upon the assumption that costs should be charged in the order in which they occur. Therefore, the remaining inventory is assumed to be based upon the most recent cost incurred. Using the foregoing data for the IV solution, and assuming that the inventory is composed of the most recent costs, the cost of the remaining case is $22. But what if two cases remain on hand at the end of the year? By using FIFO, the cost of the remaining units is determined as follows:

Most recent cost, 9/30/80:   1 case at $22 = $22
Next most recent cost, 5/30/80:   1 case at $18 = $18
Inventory: 2 cases   = $40

In general, FIFO is the most acceptable method of inventory accounting because it is in general harmony with the physical movement of issues, assuming that a good stock rotation policy exists.

Last In, First Out

The last in, first out (LIFO) method assumes that the most recent costs incurred should be charged to the issue. The remaining inventory is assumed to be composed of the earliest costs. On the basis of the previous data, the cost of our IV inventory would be determined as follows:

One case remaining in inventory—

Earliest cost, 1/1/80:   1 case at $18 = $18

Two cases remaining in inventory—

Earliest cost, 1/1/80:   1 case at $18 = $18
Net earliest cost, 2/27/80:   1 case at $18 = $18
Inventory: 2 cases   = $36

Weighted Average

The weighted average method assumes that the cost should be charged on the basis of the average, taking into consideration the number of units purchased at each price. The average unit cost is used in calculating the cost of the remaining inventory. The weighted average is determined by dividing the total cost of the item by the total number of units available for issue. On the basis of the previous data, the cost of our IV inventory would be determined as follows:

One case remaining in inventory—

Weighted average cost: $76 ÷ 4 cases = $19 per case
Inventory: 1 case at $19 = $19

Two cases remaining in inventory—

Weighted average cost: $76 ÷ 4 cases = $19 per case
Inventory: 2 cases at $19 = $38

Comparison of Inventory Costing Methods

As previously noted, each of these methods is based on a different assumption as to the flow of costs. If the unit price for our IV solution remained the same throughout the year, all of these methods would yield the same results. The data used for our IV solution show the effect of rising prices and the effects on ending inventory. They can be summarized as follows:

Ending Inventory	FIFO	LIFO	Weighted Average
1 case	$22	$18	$19
2 cases	$40	$36	$38

Inventory costing methods not only affect ending inventory, but they also affect total dollars issued. Their results can be as dramatic as their impact on ending inventory.

Using FIFO, total issues for the IV solution data are calculated as follows:

	Cases	Total Cost
Amount available for issue	4	$76
Remaining inventory	1	$22
Cost of issues		$54

Using LIFO for the same data:

	Cases	Total Cost
Amount available for issue	4	$76
Remaining inventory	1	$18
Cost of issues		$58

Using weighted average, the same data yield:

	Cases	Total Cost
Amount available for issue	4	$76
Remaining inventory	1	$19
Cost of issues		$57

Summarizing both ending inventory and cost of issues shows:

	FIFO	LIFO	Weighted Average
Amount available for issue	$76	$76	$76
Remaining inventory (one case)	$22	$18	$19
Cost of issues	$54	$58	$57

The results of the total comparison for our example show that:

- FIFO yields the highest ending inventory and lowest cost of total issues.

- LIFO yields the lowest ending·inventory and the highest cost of total issues.

- Weighted average is a compromise between FIFO and LIFO.

IMPACT ON INVENTORY SYSTEMS

Thus far, the IV solution example presented has been based upon the premise that the hospital does not utilize an inventory control system or cost accounting procedures. In reality, most hospitals use both procedures and the choice of an accounting method can and does affect both a perpetual and periodic inventory control system.

Perpetual Inventory System

Whether a hospital has a manual or computerized perpetual inventory system, FIFO is the most acceptable system to use. Again, FIFO most nearly approximates the actual flow of supplies and replacement costs. LIFO, on the other hand, does not correlate to the flow of supplies and does not reflect actual replacement costs. Weighted average is not applicable to any perpetual inventory system. The time required to gather the data is likely to be greater for the weighted average method than for FIFO or LIFO.

Periodic Control

The data used throughout our IV solution example closely approximate the results achieved if cost accounting is not utilized. Under periodic control, any of the three methods is acceptable, but the use of weighted average may not be reasonable because of the time required for the calculations.

EFFECTS OF INVENTORY ACCOUNTING

Cost Accounting Procedures

The choice of a cost determination method also extends to the costing or pricing of issues from inventory. Pricing of issues under any of the three methods is simple enough, provided, of course, that all supplies issued were purchased at the same price. However, periods of rising or declining prices tend to confuse the procedure as to price determination. Table 11-1 is used to illustrate this point.

Using the FIFO method, the illustration reflects actual cost patterns for pricing requisitions. Note that the issue of 6/10/80 for 175 units reflects a proper breakdown of cost per unit (150 units at $1.00 + 25 units at $1.10).

Now let us assume that the LIFO method of calculation is being used. The figures shown through 3/1/80 remain the same. The issue of 6/10/80 would be priced as follows: 50 units at $1.10 and 125 units at $1.00 equalling $180. The inventory balance would also reflect a reduction of on-hand balance to 25 units at $1.

The important point here is to reflect accurately the actual unit price for each item issued. Too often, inventory issues are posted at the latest unit price regardless of what the item cost. Depending upon the method used, the requisition could reflect either an over- or understatement of actual costs.

Patient Charge Supplies

In some hospitals, practitioners are responsible for adjusting patient charges to reflect changes in unit cost. Typically, patient charges are the result of marking up unit costs by a specific percentage. For example, an item with a unit cost of $1 and a markup of 200 percent equals a patient charge of $2. Recognizing that the manner in which markups are determined will vary by as many hospitals as there are throughout the country, we note that the method used to determine the cost of inventory will have a corresponding effect on revenue.

During periods of consistently rising prices, the use of FIFO yields the highest gross income. The reason for this effect is that hospitals tend to raise charges in accordance with market trends, regardless of the fact that items in stock may have been purchased prior to the price increase. In periods of declining prices, the effect is reversed, and the FIFO method yields the lowest possible gross income. The principal criticism of the FIFO method is that it tends to accentuate the effect of inflationary and deflationary trends in gross income.

During periods of consistently rising prices, the use of LIFO yields the lowest possible amount of gross income. The reason is that the cost of the most recently acquired units most nearly approximates the expenditures required to replace units issued. In periods of declining prices, the effect is reversed and the LIFO method

Table 11-1 Inventory Record

DATE	PURCHASES QTY	PURCHASES TOTAL COST	ISSUES QTY	ISSUES TOTAL COST	INVENTORY BALANCE QTY	INVENTORY BALANCE TOTAL COST	INVENTORY BALANCE UNIT COST
1/1/80					100	$ 100.00	$ 1.00
2/3/80	100	$ 100			200	200.00	1.00
2/5/80			50	$ 50	150	150.00	1.00
3/1/80	50	55			150	150.00	1.00
					50	55.00	1.10
6/10/80			175	177.50	25	27.50	1.10
7/1/80	150	165			175	192.50	1.10

yields the highest possible gross income. The main criticism of LIFO is its complete lack of any relationship to the physical flow of merchandise. The amount reported for inventory on the hospital balance sheet may also be quite removed from current replacement costs. If there is little change in the physical composition of the inventory from year to year, the inventory costs reported remain constant, regardless of extensive changes in price levels.

INVENTORY ACCOUNTING RECORDS

An important part of inventory accounting is the maintenance of accurate records relative to monthly and annual inventory dollar activity. This task can be accomplished through the establishment of a balance sheet, an issue history summary, and a purchase history summary. These records will provide the inventory manager with the information necessary to develop a meaningful analysis of the total inventory activity.

Balance Sheet

An inventory balance sheet is the principal accounting statement for the inventory. It is a summary in dollars of activity relative to purchases, issues, returns, and other changes (shrinkage/obsolescence, etc.) that take place during a specific time period. Assuming that a cost accounting system is in use, Table 11-2 illustrates a typical inventory balance sheet. As you will note, each specific inventory classification has its own section, with a summary of the total activity at the bottom of the page.

Inventory balance sheets are typically maintained on a monthly basis by fiscal year. Such a balance sheet can be used for comparison against previous years, quarters, or months. Analysis of the balance sheet by specific time periods is useful for forecasting budgets, cash flow, or future time periods.

All figures for the balance sheet are obtained from other reports generated either in accounting or central stores. Beginning inventory for the first month of the fiscal year is a restatement of the closing balance of the physical inventory taken at the close of the previous fiscal year.

Purchases are the result of those invoices processed by accounts payable during the period. The dollar figure for purchases is really only a reflection of part of the dollars actually received. Practitioners should recognize that accounts payable will not process all of the invoices for items received during the period. It is a fact of life that accounts payable will always be behind with invoice processing, and will not catch up with the workload until the end of the fiscal year. Therefore, the dollar figure on the accounts payable register should be used as a guide or, at best, an estimate. The numbers will be close, but not accurate to the penny.

Table 11-2 Inventory Balance Sheet

CENTRAL STORES INVENTORY 1980

	January	February	March	April	May
Administrative					
Beginning Inventory	44,363.88	43,875.13	38,168.40	37,474.64	38,721.71
Purchases (+)	10,658.03	5,815.86	10,359.57	12,580.14	19,568.07
Issues (−)	11,146.78	11,522.59	11,053.33	11,333.07	10,817.30
Adjustments (+/−)					
Ending Inventory	43,875.13	38,168.40	37,474.64	38,721.71	47,472.48
Housekeeping Supplies					
Beginning Inventory	6,072.77	6,593.80	5,175.12	5,854.51	5,108.44
Purchases (+)	6,484.36	5,368.55	6,928.91	6,902.71	6,876.92
Issues (−)	5,963.33	6,787.23	6,249.52	7,648.78	5,276.84
Adjustments (+/−)					
Ending Inventory	6,593.80	5,175.12	5,854.51	5,108.44	6,708.52
Medical/Surgical Supplies					
Beginning Inventory	88,810.75	89,614.96	65,268.20	71,233.32	68,002.94
Purchases (+)	64,376.44	60,076.43	75,029.61	85,937.14	88,168.06
Issues (−)	63,572.23	84,423.19	69,064.49	89,167.52	77,078.19
Adjustments (+/−)					
Ending Inventory	89,614.96	65,268.20	71,233.32	68,002.94	79,092.81
Total Ending Inventory	140,083.89	108,611.72	114,562.47	111,833.09	133,273.81

The issue figure is the summation of all requisitions processed by the storeroom during the period. This figure should be exact—which brings up an important question as to who prices stores requisitions in hospitals without a computerized inventory. In some hospitals, accounting personnel are responsible for pricing stores requisitions. In others, inventory or stores personnel price requisitions. The preferred method for the practitioner should be to have inventory or stores personnel price all requisitions, primarily because in too many instances, accounting never seems to have time to keep unit prices up to date. In one hospital where accounting priced requisitions, the ending inventory never balanced with the figures accounting maintained. The physical inventory figure was always lower than accounting's figure for ending inventory. Investigation revealed that accounting was using prices that were three years old and had never been updated. Admittedly, this situation may not be applicable to every hospital— but it does reflect what could happen.

Another reason for using inventory personnel is that they should have access to current pricing and inventory balances. Stores personnel are as responsible for inventory management as is the inventory manager and should, therefore, maintain consistency in that responsibility.

It should also be pointed out that the use of stores personnel to price requisitions violates the concept of a checks and balances system. Many accounting people believe that requisitions can be falsified. Under a manual system, this is a real possibility, and even with a computerized system falsification of requisitions is possible. But the checks and balances system can be maintained by establishing routine audit procedures to review requisitions to determine their validity and accuracy. For practitioners and accounting personnel who are skeptical of this procedure, this author has successfully utilized this procedure for over six years in two hospitals without an incident of falsification.

Returns to the inventory are simply that, returns. Maintaining this figure has proved especially useful in demonstrating savings of excessive inventory removed during the implementation of PAR level, exchange cart, or special departmental control procedures. This is an optional category inasmuch as returns can be credited against issues.

The line used to reflect changes simply summarizes shrinkage/obsolescence that is discovered during the period. Maintaining this figure has proved useful in identifying trends in losses to inventory. Should a trend appear, it is an automatic signal that something is wrong, either with the system or the procedure.

Issue and Purchase Summary

Separate summaries of issues and purchases by month and year to date are also recommended (see Tables 11-3 and 11-4). These two records are used in tracking trends and forecasting future activity. Changes that occur from year to year are compared with purchase price index results (Chapter 13) to discern general changes in usage relative to the effects of rising or declining prices. Again, these figures are total figures and are not specific to any particular department. Dramatic increases or decreases in either of the figures usually trigger further specific investigation to determine and test for probable causes. Maintaining separate summary information for issues also saves time in calculating turnover rates, days of inventory, and dollars per bed as discussed in the preceding chapter.

INVENTORY AUDITING

Internal inventory auditing is a procedure that is necessary to ensure that the proper controls are in place with regard to inventory management. Normally, inventory auditing is accomplished by the hospital's auditing firm or the account-

Table 11-3 Total Issues Summary

CENTRAL STORES INVENTORY 1980
TOTAL ISSUES SUMMARY

Month	Administrative	Housekeeping	Medical/Surgical	Total
January	11,146.78	5,963.33	63,572.23	80,682.34
February	11,522.59	6,787.23	84,423.19	102,733.01
March	11,053.33	6,249.52	69,064.49	86,367.34
April	11,333.07	7,648.78	89,167.52	108,149.37
May	10,817.30	5,276.84	77,078.19	93,172.33
June	8,746.74	6,629.18	78,785.41	94,161.33
July	10,434.29	6,907.10	83,082.25	100,423.64
August	11,869.33	6,359.54	80,255.46	98,484.33
September	14,840.58	8,871.60	104,884.62	128,596.80
October	13,063.75	7,025.73	87,088.70	107,177.68
November	9,651.13	5,619.77	80,080.54	95,351.44
December	18,469.82	8,232.67	77,047.82	103,750.31
1980 YEAR-TO-DATE SUMMARY				
January	11,146.78	5,963.33	63,572.23	80,682.34
February	22,669.37	12,750.56	147,995.42	183,415.35
March	33,722.70	19,000.08	217,059.91	269.782.69
April	45,055.77	26,648.86	306,227.43	377,932.06
May	55,873.07	31,925.70	383,305.62	471,104.39
June	64,619.81	38,554.88	462,091.03	565,265.72
July	75,054.10	45,461.98	545,173.28	665,689.36
August	86,923.43	51,821.52	625,428.74	764,173.69
September	101,764.01	60,693.12	730,313.36	892,770.49
October	114,827.76	67,718.85	817,401.56	999,948.17
November	124,478.89	73,338.62	897,482.10	1,095,299.61
December	142,948.71	81,571.29	974,529.92	1,199,049.92

ing department. These audits generally are conducted on an annual basis and usually are just a cursory look at the inventory management program. Unless some major discrepancies are discovered, this procedure usually suffices to meet required review criteria. However, the fact remains that the inventory manager holds the ultimate responsibility to ensure that the necessary controls are in place and properly functioning. Therefore, it is important that the inventory manager understand the auditing procedures necessary to accomplish this.

How is an effective inventory auditing procedure established? Such procedures must begin by answering what is to be audited first, and the how questions will fall naturally into place. The thrust of inventory auditing should be in the areas of inventory records versus actual physical counts; pricing of requisitions under a manual system; issues of material to proper using departments; proper processing of patient charges; inventory pricing practices; etc.

Table 11-4 Total Purchases Summary

CENTRAL STORES INVENTORY 1980
TOTAL PURCHASES SUMMARY

Month	Administrative	Housekeeping	Medical/Surgical	Total
January	10,658.03	6,484.36	64,376.44	81,518.83
February	5,815.86	5,368.55	60,076.43	71,260.84
March	10,359.57	6,928.91	75,029.61	92,318.09
April	12,580.14	6,902.71	85,937.14	105,419.99
May	19,568.07	6,876.92	88,168.06	114,613.05
June	17,405.97	12,139.09	103,102.97	132,648.03
July	9,273.29	4,657.18	71,979.15	85,909.62
August	5,014.50	8,206.84	69,542.99	82,764.33
September	8,324.99	7,202.77	94,298.74	109,826.50
October	20,712.60	8,981.38	133,904.87	163,598.85
November	6,018.45	9,488.58	57,347.06	72,854.09
December	16,025.45	6,905.98	131,411.77	154,343.20
1980 YEAR-TO-DATE SUMMARY				
January	10,658.03	6,484.36	64,376.44	81,518.83
February	16,473.89	11,852.91	124,452.87	152,779.67
March	26,833.46	18,781.82	199,482.48	245,097.76
April	39,413.60	25,684.53	285,419.62	350,517.75
May	58,981.67	32,561.45	373,587.68	465,130.80
June	76,387.64	44,700.54	476,690.65	597,778.83
July	85,660.93	49,357.72	548,669.80	683,688.45
August	90,675.43	57,564.56	618,212.79	766,452.78
September	99,000.42	64,767.33	712,511.53	876,279.28
October	119,713.02	73,748.71	846,416.40	1,039,878.13
November	125,731.47	83,237.29	903,763.46	1,112,732.22
December	141,756.72	90,143.27	1,035,243.80	1,267,143.99

The actual auditing procedures will vary by what it is you are attempting to audit. Before you can attempt to audit any part of the system, a clearly established objective must be defined. Once the objective is defined, the audit steps necessary to accomplish the objective must be outlined. This is the how-to portion of the procedure. To enable the reader to understand this process better, an actual example is provided with Exhibit 11-1.

With this example, it is important to note that the systematic audit for pricing requisitions reflects auditing pricing back through the actual invoice pricing. This procedure is necessary to verify that the same costs are reflected throughout the system. Consistency is the key to ensuring that the entire system reflects identical information.

Exhibit 11-1 Audit Procedure

Objective: To determine if inventory requisitions are properly priced.

Audit Steps:

1. Select a number of supply requisitions for each inventory category for a specific time period.
2. Compare the quantities for each line item on the requisition with the inventory record postings.
3. Compare the unit pricing for each requisition line item with the pricing maintained on the individual inventory record.
4. Compare the unit pricing for each inventory record with the appropriate corresponding purchase cost. (Recognize that changes in purchase cost may have occurred during the period. Check to see that if a change has occurred, the inventory records were properly updated to reflect the change.)
5. Compare the latest invoice costs with the purchase costs for the appropriate time period involved.

The logic applied to the requisition pricing example should be consistently applied to other areas that can be audited. The important points to be remembered when setting up an audit procedure are:

1. Establish a clear objective to be achieved.
2. Establish a step-by-step logical process to acquire and examine the information.
3. Evaluate the information in terms of success or failure in achieving the objective.
4. Communicate the results of the audit to the appropriate managers with appropriate recommendations to correct any deficiencies that exist.

Chapter 12

Supply Storage
and Distribution

Historically, practitioners have complained of a lack of adequate storage space
in which to maintain the inventory level required to meet the demands of the
hospital. In a majority of cases, the practitioner's complaints have fallen on deaf
ears. In other cases, administrators have sympathy for the practitioner's plight, but
are unable to provide additional space owing to the physical constraints of existing
facilities. In hospitals considering expansion, additional storage space for central
stores is most often at the bottom of the priority list in deference to the needs for
expanded patient care services. Only in a few cases is the question of additional
storage space considered in hospital expansion plans.

Given these circumstances, practitioners must become creative and improve
utilization of the space currently available. Therefore, in this chapter we deal with
the problem of storage on the basis of working within the confines of existing
space.

Closely associated with space considerations is the subject of supply distribution. The movement and control of supplies throughout the hospital are   major
concerns for practitioners. Later in this chapter, we look at the alternatives available
for a modern supply distribution program.

FACILITY PLANNING

Any plan for maximizing storage space must begin by identifying the physical
requirements for every item to be stored within the given space. This identification
process requires that every item be categorized by size, shape, and weight for the
maximum amount of inventory. The information thus gleaned is used to identify
the type of storage required, that is, box, shelf, or pallet. Items are then sorted by
storage requirements to determine an accurate picture of the total requirements for
each type of storage unit. For example, all items requiring pallet storage are

205

grouped together. Individual item analysis must also include total cubic requirements. Once this information is complete, you are ready to move to the next phase of the planning process.

The design and layout process starts by defining the physical dimensions of the storage area, including ceiling height, room dimensions, location of support columns, and lighting arrangement. In many cases, the maintenance department will have scale blueprints of the area for your use. If blueprints are not available, it may be necessary to measure the area and create your own scale drawings. If it is necessary to create your own drawings, a scale of one-quarter inch to one foot is recommended. Quarter-inch scale provides the best space perception.

Once the room drawings are completed, templates should be made in the same scale to represent existing shelving units and pallets. Shelving templates should identify the number of shelves per unit; templates can serve as aisles.

At this point, it is important to review types of storage units. Shelves are available in various widths, lengths, and heights. They should be selected on the basis of the type of item to be stored. Depths of 12, 18, and 24 inches are the most popular and appropriate sizes for use in a storeroom. Weight bearing capabilities should also be considered, as should use and type of pallets. Metal pallets are the ideal, whereas wooden pallets, which do present fire hazards, are cheaper.

Once the templates are completed, all logical layouts should be considered. Layouts can be based on the use of static shelving or an active aisle system. A static layout utilizes straight lines with uniform shelving arrangements for maximum accessibility and orderly flow of materials. Figure 12-1 illustrates the static aisle concept. Notice that this arrangement accommodates an orderly flow of material from the receiving area to storage, and from storage to the user. The main traffic aisle is wide enough to accommodate various types of material-handling equipment. The stocking and picking aisles that radiate from the traffic aisle are narrower. These aisles may vary in width to accommodate the various sizes and volumes of the material stored in the location.

An alternative to the static layout is a storage concept known as active aisle. The active aisle concept utilizes movable carts on tracks with the aisles created by the movement of the carts (Figure 12-2). This concept tends to maximize available square footage that is normally lost to required aisles in the static concept. The manufacturers of active aisle systems claim improved utilization of floor space by more than 50 percent. Such claims may be true in some cases, but practitioners considering this type of storage should compare the actual difference between the amount of shelf space available with the active aisle system versus that available with the current or proposed static shelving. This author's experience with active aisle showed an increase of 40 percent for available shelf space in a very small storeroom. Active aisle also helped to facilitate traffic flow in this case. Any improvements will depend upon current available square footage, room design, and the amount of available static shelving. Active aisle is a sound concept when

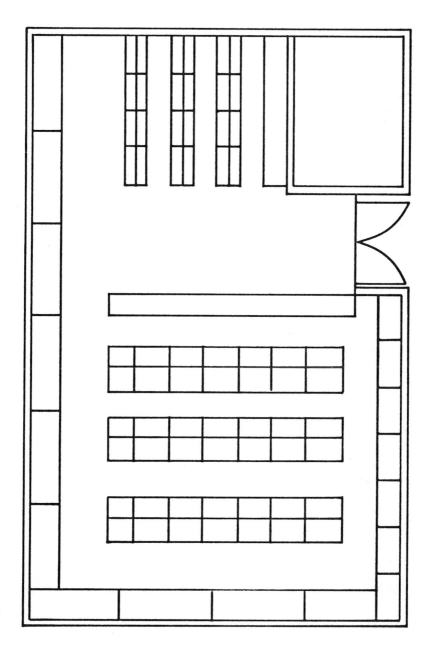

Figure 12-1 Static Aisle Concept

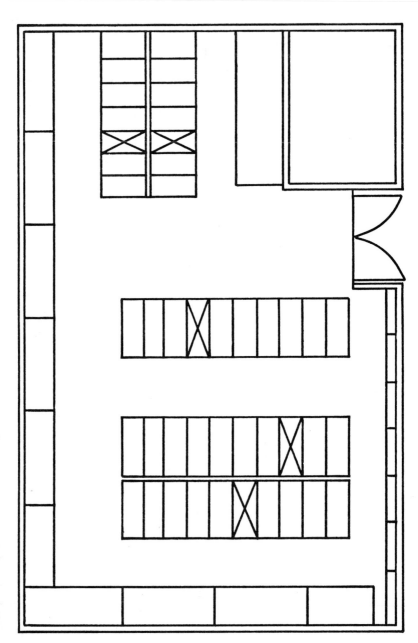

Figure 12-2 Active Aisle Concept

employed for loose issue items, but is impractical for heavy bulk storage. Active aisle also is very expensive, and practitioners should review any proposals with the idea of determining where the payback will come from.

Finally, a properly designed storeroom not only considers maximum use of available floor space, but also maximizes the use of available cubic space. Maximizing cubic space is often forgotten during the design stage. Individual item storage must take into consideration upward as well as horizontal storage. A rule of thumb that has been found useful is: to maximize storage space think upward; don't spread it out.

Physical Requirements

Every storeroom has its physical limitations that extend beyond size to type of floors, walls, ceilings, lighting, etc. For the practitioner, these characteristics are as important as available square footage.

Floors in a storeroom should be sealed concrete. Terrazzo or vinyl tile floors look good, but are impractical to maintain.

Walls should also be concrete or concrete block. They should be painted a bright, cheerful color. Nothing is more depressing in a storeroom than gray walls.

Ceiling height should be at least 8 to 10 feet clear height (floor to bottom of light fixtures or sprinklers); anything less will limit the available cubic space. Ceiling height will also be a limiting factor on the height of shelving units. If the current area has an open ceiling, provisions for continued housekeeping will be necessary. Open ceilings create an excessive amount of dirt, especially if there are concrete floors above.

Lighting can be another physical limitation. Lighting patterns should be adequate to prevent dark areas in aisles. Storeroom personnel cannot pick items they cannot see. Practitioners should also be aware that NFPA fire codes require that upward storage must be maintained at a minimum of 18 inches below lighting fixtures, ceilings, or sprinkler heads.

Stock Locations

Every storage facility should have a stock location system in order to prevent lost motion and delays in locating inventory items. A definite address for every stock item is necessary to maintain order, efficient storage, and order filling. A simple, efficient location system of labeling shelving and pallets can be accomplished by using letters, numbers, or a combination of both. A complete location system also includes a file or catalog maintained either in stock number sequence or alphabetically with location codes. Remember, this record must also be current and changes should be posted as soon as they occur.

Materials should be stored or located in relation to their proximity to receiving and issuing areas. Typically, items are stored on the basis of popularity, similarity, size, or characteristics.

Storage based upon popularity refers to frequency of demand, and usually coincides with the ABC concept. With this storage methodology, popular A items are stored closest to the major traffic aisle or work area. Medium B movers are next, followed by slow-moving C items, which are last or furthest from the traffic aisle or work area. This methodology assumes that a majority of stocking and issuing activity will be completed near the work area and limits the average travel time for the work to be accomplished. Storage by popularity should be the first consideration.

Storage based upon similarity refers to items that are frequently ordered or used by one department and are stored close to each other to avoid unnecessary travel between items. For example, items used and ordered frequently by surgery would be stocked in the same area. Storage by similarity should be second to popularity.

Storage based upon size is the third possibility. Its size will influence how an item will be stored. Adequate space must be provided to balance the inventory requirements with the need for maximum space utilization. Both can be met by minimizing the height of shelves above stock located on the shelf below.

Storage based upon characteristics refers to those items that cannot or should not be stored on the basis of the previously mentioned possibilities. For example, perishable items require storage in a refrigerator or freezer; needles and syringes may require storage in a security area; and hazardous or toxic items will require storage in a special room designed for such items.

Equipment Selection

Equipment requirements should be based upon:

- material to be handled (type, size, weight)

- volume to be handled and number of times movement will occur

- distance material will be moved

- physical limitations: ceiling height, floor loads, inclines of ramps, elevator weight restrictions, etc.

- available equipment that is currently in use and equipment that is available but not being used

- safety requirements to prevent accidents or injury to employees using the equipment

Equipment selection requires analysis to meet the functional requirements associated with proper material handling. Every effort should be made to combine or eliminate operations to reduce handling. Equipment should be selected that will aid in eliminating delays due to congestion. Maintenance of the required quantity of an equipment type will also aid in reducing congestion and unproductive time caused by a lack of available equipment.

The types of equipment used in a storeroom include, but are not limited to:

- *Platform trucks,* used primarily for movement of large quantities of boxes, packages, etc. Platform trucks are available with steel or wooden decks. Sizes range from 24 inches wide by 42 inches long to 30 inches wide by 60 inches long; weight capacity from 1000 to 3000 pounds. Cost is $130 to $250.

- *Two-wheel hand trucks,* used primarily for movement of case stock, and loading and unloading delivery vehicles. Weight capacity ranges from 450 to 1000 pounds. Cost is $50 to $130.

- *Drum truck,* used primarily for loading, unloading, and transportation of barrels and drums. Available in two- or four-wheel models. Weight capacity is up to 1000 pounds. Cost is $100 to $300.

- *Oxygen tank trucks.* Movement of cylinders is the primary purpose of this special design equipment. Capacity will vary from one or two "H" cylinders to four "E" cylinders. Cost is $50 to $125.

- *Appliance hand truck.* Design is similar to general-purpose two-wheel truck except that this vehicle can be used to move refrigerators, file cabinets, and other large pieces of furniture safely. Weight capacity is 200 to 1000 pounds. Cost is $100 to $200.

- *Platform dolly,* designed to move equipment, furniture, refrigerators, etc. Can be made from oak or steel with varying caster sizes. Weight capacity is 800 to 2000 pounds. Cost is $25 to $50.

- *Hand pallet truck,* designed specifically to move wooden or metal pallets. Manufactured with varying widths from 20 to 27 inches, and lengths from 32 to 48 inches. Weight capacities range from 2000 to 6000 pounds per load. Cost is $400 to $600.

SUPPLY DISTRIBUTION

The problems associated with a well-planned storage facility extend beyond the wall of the storeroom. Up to now we have limited the discussion of inventory management to those items maintained within the storeroom. A logical extension of inventory management is supply distribution.

The increased popularity of the materiel management concept has broadened the scope of inventory management to extend to the nursing units and other departments. These other departments have traditionally been off limits to the practitioner, but the advent of materiel management is removing the obstacles to extended inventory management. This extension brings with it the need for the practitioner to review and update the methods of supply distribution.

Hospital supply distribution consists of five basic methodologies: direct requisition, fetch and carry, PAR level, exchange cart, and stockless inventory programs. Both PAR level and exchange cart are variations of the same procedure.

Direct Requisition

The direct requisition procedure is the oldest and most traditional method used by hospitals. With this procedure, each department determines its own needs. The order is transmitted to the storeroom, where it is filled and delivered to the department. Depending upon the nature of the item, the requisition is charged either to the department or to the patient. Exhibit 12-1 represents a standard requisition form.

The use of direct requisitions creates a second inventory for storeroom items, one in stores and the other in the user department. As noted in Chapter 11, one inventory is official (stores) and the second (user) is unofficial. Regardless of how the second inventory is accounted for by accounting, it is usually controlled in relation to the department's comfort factor. A comfort factor is the feeling the department has for the storeroom's ability to supply the item upon demand. The consistency of performance by the storeroom will be the deciding or influencing item that determines if the comfort factor is high or low. A low comfort factor will cause the using department to maintain higher levels of supplies, in case the storeroom runs out. But a high comfort factor does not necessarily produce the reverse effect. Users will continue to maintain traditional levels in the event a stock-out occurs in the storeroom.

The effect of the user comfort factor usually results in excessive inventory being maintained within the user's department. To many practitioners, excessive really means hoarding. As a practitioner, this author can appreciate the user's feelings for maintaining excessive inventory. Some practitioners may infer that this statement supports this practice. Be assured that it does not. If excessive inventory is being maintained by the user, the reason is the storeroom's failure to support the requirements of the user. Granted, this is not always the case. All of us at one time or another have heard stories of ten years' worth of autopsy reports being maintained on the nursing units, or something similar. The blame for excessive inventory is a two-way street. If you want the users to reduce inventory, prove to them that their requirements can be supported by the storeroom.

Exhibit 12-1 Storeroom Requisition

ST. FRANCIS HOSPITAL
BLUE ISLAND, ILL.

REQUISITION
FOR SUPPLIES

DATE:

DEPARTMENT:

APPROVED BY:

STOCK NO.	UNIT OF ISSUE	QUANTITY ORDERED	RCD. √	UNIT COST	TOTAL

DO NOT WRITE IN THESE COLUMNS

RECEIVED BY:

DATE:

TOTALS

ADM.
HSKP.
M & S
TOTAL

21-05

FETCH AND CARRY

The fetch and carry procedure is a variation of the direct requisition procedure. The difference is in the delivery method. With the fetch and carry procedure, the user prepares a direct requisition, hand carries it to the storeroom, picks up the material, and returns with it to the department.

This procedure normally is followed by the requesting department when the material is required for immediate use and the need is such that it will not wait for delivery of the order by storeroom personnel.

This procedure can also be adopted as a normal routine for obtaining supplies. The problems of excessive unofficial inventory described under the direct requisition procedure are applicable to this procedure as well. The fetch and carry method also contributes to the loss of productive time in the user departments. That is, user department personnel may be required to spend more time traveling to and from the storeroom than in accomplishing the work they were originally hired to do.

PAR LEVEL

PAR level programs involve working with the user to establish standard maximum quantities for both patient charge and unit charge supply items. Traditional PAR programs utilize existing shelving or cabinets within the department. Supplies are checked periodically by storeroom personnel and refilled to bring each item up to the established standard. The frequency of replenishment is a variable that can be adjusted to meet the specific requirements of the user. For example, a PAR program on a nursing unit may require daily replenishment, whereas a PAR program in radiology may require weekly replenishment. The important point is to determine with the user a reasonable schedule that will accommodate the needs of both departments.

The establishment of a PAR level program should accomplish two objectives. The first is to bring user department inventories under the control of one central inventory manager. The second objective is to take the user department out of the supply business; that is, to eliminate user department personnel for the functions of requisitioning, inventory management, etc.

Proposed implementation of a PAR level program usually invokes extreme reactions from the user departments. Those departments who really dislike controlling their department inventory will welcome the program with open arms. Experience has shown, at least to this author, that departments that welcome the idea usually are the departments that are doing a credible job of inventory management. That is not to say that departments that are not pleased with the idea of a PAR program are the ones doing a poor job. Their objections usually arise from a feeling of invasion of established domain and that such a program is a threat to the operation in the form of increased potential for stock-outs. Approaching these departments and gaining their trust require both patience and tact. Here, the soft sell approach is often successful. The department's confidence is gained by establishing liberal maximums and working extra hard to make sure there are few, if any, stock-outs. Then, once a good track record is established, maximum levels are gradually reduced to levels that are realistic. This process usually takes six months to achieve, but it does work. This approach has been criticized because inventory reduction is not achieved immediately. While that criticism is true, it should also be remembered that the excessive inventory has existed for years. So what is another six months as long as the objective is ultimately achieved?

Establishment of a PAR level program will present the opportunity to bring unofficial inventory into the official classification. When this occurs, official inventory dollars will begin to go up until excessive stocks are used up. When a department is converted to a PAR program, the department should receive credit for all existing inventory. Determining when the items were withdrawn from the storeroom will be an almost impossible task. Therefore, as a practical matter, credit should be based on the latest cost of inventory. Later issue of the material will also be charged out at the latest cost, so it will even out eventually. Credit should only be given for items that can be reissued. Any item that appears to be unusable should be thrown out.

During the conversion process it is also recommended that "other" storage areas be checked for backup supplies. This includes all drawers and cabinets throughout the department. User departments are creative in storing backup supplies. For example, at one hospital the second and third shifts had their own stock of flashlight batteries and ballpoint pens stored in the drop ceiling in the nurses' station.

Establishing a PAR level program for any department will be subject to the physical constraints of available shelving/cabinetry. The following guidelines should be followed as closely as possible when establishing the location of supplies for this program:

- Generically similar items should be stored together, that is, all tapes, I.V. supplies, etc.

- High-usage A and B items should be placed between waist and eye level to permit easy access and location by user department personnel.

- Bulk items (bedpans, admission kits, etc.) should be nearer the floor.

- Low usage C items should be placed toward the top of the cabinet/shelving unit, or at the back of the unit when combined with the first two categories listed.

Supplemental to the foregoing procedures is the need to work closely with the department head in establishing stock locations. Usage determination (ABC) is not based on storeroom usage, but on user usage and the fact that departmental personnel must identify stock locations quickly. Flexibility in location of stock is a paramount consideration for the success of this program.

As a final note on PAR level, the major drawback to this distribution system is the actual replenishment of stock. This can be achieved through either of two procedures. The first is to have stores personnel inventory each department, return to the storeroom, draw the necessary stock, and return to the unit. The second procedure is to replenish common supplies from a master cart.

The first procedure usually results in some items not being brought up to the established standard. This will happen because the user continues to draw from the inventory during the time stores personnel is drawing stock from the storeroom.

The master cart alternative is usually more effective, except that it is not always possible to carry adequate stock on the cart to meet the needs of all the nursing units.

Both options should be evaluated and the best solution chosen for the particular hospital.

Another problem that arises with either of these methods is that storeroom personnel must be away from their department for extended periods of time. They usually like this situation because it gives them an opportunity to visit other areas of the hospital, but it also means that unproductive time may increase dramatically if left uncontrolled.

EXCHANGE CART

An exchange cart program can be equated to a PAR level program on wheels. The approach to the exchange cart is basically the same as the PAR program. The requisition form used for both is shown in Exhibit 12-2.

Initially, exchange cart programs require fairly large investments, with a typical cart costing $400 or more.

Although the number will vary, the minimum requirement is two carts per user department. One cart is stored on the unit and the second identically stocked cart is maintained in the storeroom. The normal procedure is to take the full cart from the storeroom and return the depleted cart at a predetermined time every day. The depleted cart is then restocked and readied for delivery the next day.

Exchange cart programs appear to be the most efficient method of supply distribution available. Stores personnel spend most of their time in the storeroom because the actual exchange time is minimal, thus improving productivity because they have more time to complete other tasks. Quality control is improved because carts can be checked prior to storage for the next day's exchange. A quality control

Exhibit 12-2 PAR or Exchange Cart Requisition

ST. FRANCIS HOSPITAL
BLUE ISLAND, ILLINOIS

CENTRAL SERVICE REQUISITION

NURSING UNIT _____   WEEK OF _____

STOCK NR.	ITEM DESCRIPTION	PAR	ISSUES							TOTAL	UNIT COST	TOTAL COST
			S	M	TU	W	TH	F	ST			

program is necessary to assure user departments that established standards are being met on the full cart.

Exchange carts traditionally are used to distribute medical/surgical supplies and linen to the nursing units. In some instances, surgery, emergency room, and physical therapy can be converted to an exchange cart program. The only limitations of an exchange cart program are those placed on it by the practitioner and the physical layout of the hospital.

The location of stock on the exchange cart should follow the guidelines established for the PAR level program. Again, user participation in establishing stock locations is an important part of the program.

With most cart exchange programs, either the user can draw from both sides of the cart, or only from a single side. The two-sided system limits the physical quantity of stock that can be maintained for each line item. However, it does permit improved visibility of lower usage C items.

The one-sided draw system allows for a larger quantity of items, but presents a disadvantage in that lower usage C items tend to be maintained toward the back of the cart, where they are more difficult to find. In addition, stores personnel tend to "overlook" items normally kept on the back of the shelf, and so such items may not be replenished as necessary. For this reason, a sound quality control system should be implemented to ensure that all items required on the cart are there.

STOCKLESS INVENTORY

Up to this point, our discussion has centered around supply distribution from the storeroom. As a supply distribution method, stockless inventory represents an alternative to maintaining supplies in the storeroom.

Stockless inventory is aimed at those items that are used primarily by only one or two departments. Specifically, departments such as laboratory, radiology, surgery, and other specialized departments are ideally suited for a program of stockless inventory.

Stockless inventory management is accomplished by identifying specialized departmental supplies, establishing appropriate departmental inventory quotas, and processing orders for these supplies directly to the user department without accumulating an inventory in the storeroom. The primary objective of stockless inventory management is to establish and maintain limited specified quantities of unofficial inventory.

Establishing a stockless inventory program begins by identifying those storeroom items being maintained for one or two specialized departments. These items are then combined with other nonstoreroom items for analysis of usage and supplier lead times.

Once the identification phase is completed, the next step is to sit down with the user and establish initial quotas for each item, taking into consideration usage, lead times, turnover rates, and peaks and valleys in the supply cycle. Initial quotas should be flexible so that they can be changed easily if required. Quota establishment can be based upon either the use of periodic ordering or on user departmental supply budgets. The criteria for using the budget process require dividing the user's annual supply budget by the desired number of turns per year to establish a maximum total dollar value for all items falling under the stockless inventory program.

The third and final step is to establish a routine order cycle and a special requisition to facilitate departmental ordering through the purchasing department. Ideally, the routine order cycle should allow for two orders per month. The orders should be processed on a special requisition (similar to a PAR level requisition), which identifies each specific line item, the established maximum quota, and the quantity required to bring stock up to that quota.

A stockless inventory management program offers many advantages, including:

- It allows more efficient utilization of the storeroom by freeing valuable space.

- Inventory holding costs are reduced because there is less stock on hand.

- The elimination of one level of supply duplication primarily in the storeroom enables the hospital to save money through inventory reduction.

- Maintenance of a stockless inventory places greater responsibility on the department head for increased effective supply utilization and cost containment.

- A reduction in inventory shrinkage should be accomplished.

- The system provides for more control over unofficial inventories.

Stockless inventory should not be viewed as a sure way to obtain an immediate reduction in official inventory, and to "lighten" the storeroom workload. Inventory, whether official or unofficial, still requires the use of limited financial resources. Stockless inventory also requires the monitoring of user department inventories to ensure that the objectives are being met.

THE BEST PROCEDURE

The question of which procedure is best for any hospital is difficult to answer. The choice will depend on the nature of the physical plant and the economic impact of the financial resources required to establish and maintain a sound distribution program. Every consideration should be given to utilizing either a PAR level or an exchange cart, or a combination of the two.

The best combination for any hospital will be decided on the basis of the advantages and disadvantages as they exist within the facility. The important point is to centralize inventory management and supply distribution under one central manager.

Chapter 13

Price and Use Indexes

The rapid increase in hospital costs during the last two decades has been a major concern of our society. Newspapers and television carry reports seeking to determine why health care costs continue their unabated upward spirals. Recently, the federal government pointed an accusing finger at hospitals for gross inefficiency in their purchasing operations. As we all know, the blame flows down the organization chart to the purchasing practitioner.

Until recently, the purchasing practitioner had little, if any, defense or quantitative methodology to prove exactly why supply costs were rising. The two main causes for increasing costs, inflation and increased usage, have always been known. How to differentiate between the two has been the problem.

In 1979, Dean Ammer developed a quantitative methodology known as a price index to measure the effects of inflation. Exhibit 13-1 provides the basic steps in building a hospital-based price index. The Ammer price index has proved to be one of the key developments in hospital purchasing over the past five to ten years. Utilized properly, the index can provide the purchasing practitioner with a wealth of information. The discussion that follows reviews the proper methodology for a price index, introduces a new methodology for both price and use indexes, and shows how the information can be interpreted and applied to the hospital's cost database.

WHAT IS AN INDEX?

Index numbers are statistical measurements used to compare the amount of change for individual or groups of selected items. The most common indexes measure variations over periods of time versus an established base period. That is, an index will measure the difference between a current price and the price paid during a previous time period.

Exhibit 13-1 Steps To Build Hospital-Based Price Index

---

1. Pick at least 10 but no more than 50 items in each major commodity group.
2. Select a base period and prepare worksheets.
3. Regularly compare the current price of each index item with the base period.
4. Add up the percentages calculated for each item and divide by the number of items.
5. Construct composite indexes by using appropriate weight.
6. Periodically review both weights and index items.

Source: Reprinted from *Hospital Purchasing Management* by Dean S. Ammer by permission of Chi Systems, Inc., © October 30, 1980.

Indexes can be used for a variety of purposes, including the charting of trends, forecasting, inventory monitoring, efficiency measurement, and credibility. By charting index numbers a quantitative comparison can be made between activity in current periods versus activity of past periods. Use of an index system will also aid in forecasting cost during budget preparation. Inventory activity can be monitored and thus provide a basis for measuring the efficiency with which the inventory is being managed. The credibility of indexes comes into play when dealing with challenges from third party providers and state rate review commissions.

BUILDING AN INDEX

The first consideration is to determine what it is you want to measure. Indexes can be developed by specific commodity groups (x-ray film, laboratory supplies, medical/surgical supplies, etc.). Or a general "mixed" index can utilize items from each commodity or group, where you might want to measure the effects of inflation or usage on the inventory as a whole and not by specific commodity groups within the inventory. As a practical matter, indexes for specific commodity groups appear to be the best course of action. Later in this chapter, the discussion of "weighted" indexes clarifies some of the problems with mixed indexes.

The second consideration is the selection of items to measure. This can be done through random selection or by using the ABC concept. The random selection method allows for selection of any individual product for inclusion in the index without regard for annual usage, unit pricing, or manufacturer.

Use of the ABC concept as a selection process offers a number of different possibilities. One alternative is to use all A items since these items will represent 70 percent of the total dollars expended for the commodity. A second alternative would be to select items using all three classifications: 70 percent of the total number of items from the A category; 20 percent from the B category; and 10 percent from the C category. This combination affords a better overall measurement of actual activity.

Regardless of the selection process employed, care should be taken to make certain that as many different manufacturers and suppliers as possible are included in the sample. Consideration should also be given to balancing the number of items purchased through group purchasing agreements versus items purchased through competitive bidding. For example, if 40 percent of the hospital's major purchases are made through group purchasing agreements, then 40 percent of the selected items should come from this area in order accurately to reflect the total picture of the pricing structure.

The next consideration is the number of items to be included in the index. Experience has shown that ten is a good minimum figure to use. There is no ideal maximum; however, beyond 40 or 50 items the time required for the calculation becomes extensive and the difference in results appears to be negligible.

The next step is to select a base period for comparison purposes. This is an arbitrary decision that will depend on available historical data. Whenever possible, a base period that goes back two or three years should be chosen. Historical backtracking will provide a much clearer picture of what has actually transpired and a guide to establishing realistic assessments of past activities.

After establishing a base period, measurements should be made at six-month intervals to show activity trends. For example, if the fourth quarter of 1977 was chosen as the base period, measurements would be computed for the end of the second and fourth quarters for the following years until the current time period is reached. Once the data are current, routine calculations can be accomplished quarterly.

PRICE INDEX

A price index is used to measure the percentage of change in purchase price from one period to another. The standard formula for this calculation is as follows:

$$\frac{\text{Price in the Nonbase Period (PNB)}}{\text{Price in the Base Period (PB)}} \times 100 = \text{Price index}$$

To illustrate this procedure, consider item 2, "Glove, surgeon's, size 7," from Table 13-1. Substituting the given information into the formula:

$$\frac{\text{PNB}}{\text{PB}} \times 100 = \frac{17.44}{16.41} = 1.0628 \times 100 = 106.28 \text{ percent}$$

Table 13-1 Unit Price Index Worksheet for Medical/Surgical Supplies

Stock No.	Description	Unit	Base Price	Current Price	Percent Change
MB-130	Bottle, suction	40/cs	$21.50	$21.50	100.00
MG-65	Glove, surgeon's, size 7	50/bx	16.41	17.44	106.28
MH-20	Hemoclip	250/bx	44.00	75.00	170.45
MM-07	Mask, surgical	50/bx	6.248	6.614	105.86
MR-05	Razor, prep.	100/cs	27.00	25.62	94.89
MS-47	Sponge, 3 × 3	cs	74.33	82.44	110.91
MT-24	Tissues	125/bx	0.33	0.30	90.91
MT-40	Tube, endotrach., 8	each	1.97	2.07	105.08
MT-80	Tube, Yankauer	50/cs	33.00	33.00	100.00
MU-40	Underpads	150/cs	25.00	31.25	125.00
				Total	1109.38
				Divided by	10
				Index	110.94

Thus, we can conclude that a 6.28 percent price increase has occurred since the base period.

To calculate the impact of the average price change for the entire index, the following formula applies:

$$\frac{\text{Total percent change for all items}}{\text{Total number of items}} = \text{Average change}$$

Again referring to Table 13-1, you can see that the average or result of the index reflects an overall change of 10.94 percent since the base period. Also note in Table 13-1 some of the extensive variances that have occurred. Item 3, Hemoclips, shows an increase of 70.45 percent and item 7, Tissues, shows a reduction in pricing of 9.09 percent from the base period. Increases in price, such as that for Hemoclips, should be investigated to determine exactly what happened. Sometimes changes in case quantity occur and these changes will distort the index.

USE INDEX

A use index is used to measure the percentage of change in usage from one period to another. The standard formula for this calculation is:

$$\frac{\text{Quantity in the nonbase period (QNB)}}{\text{Quantity in the base period (QB)}} \times 100 = \text{Use index}$$

To illustrate this calculation, let us use the data for surgeons' gloves from Table 13-2. Substituting in the formula:

$$\frac{QNB}{QB} \times 100 = \frac{356 \text{ units}}{408 \text{ units}} = 0.8725 \times 100 = 87.25 \text{ percent}$$

Thus, we can conclude that a reduction of 12.75 percent or 52 units has occurred since the base period.

To calculate the impact of usage on the entire index, the following formula applies:

$$\frac{\text{Total percent change for all items}}{\text{Total number of items}} = \text{Average change in usage}$$

Again referring to Table 13-2, we can conclude that the usage index for medical/ surgical supplies has increased by 6.34 percent over the base period.

To some, logic would dictate that if the results of the price and use indexes were combined for our illustrations, an increase of 17.28 percent (base + price index + use index = change in total costs, or 100 + 10.94 + 6.34 = 117.28 percent) would have occurred in total costs for the same period. However, this is not the case. Table 13-3 summarizes the effects of both price and usage on the illustrated index items. You will note that when total costs are divided to determine the percentage of change, the figure equals 124.55 percent. When compared with the combined results of the price and use index noted, we discover that 117.28 does not equal 124.55. In fact, 7.22 remains unaccounted for. The problem is that we are applying index averages of what has actually occurred to total costs, without considering total costs.

Table 13-2 Usage Index Worksheet for Medical/Surgical Supplies

Stock No.	Description	Unit	Base Period	Current Period	Percent Change
MB-130	Bottle, suction	Case	216	251	116.20
MG-65	Glove, surgeon's, size 7	Box	408	356	87.25
MH-20	Hemoclips	Box	158	194	122.78
MM-07	Mask, surgical	Box	1,053	956	90.79
MR-05	Razor, prep.	Case	98	98	100.00
MS-47	Sponge, 3 × 3	Case	88	91	103.41
MT-24	Tissues	Box	12,600	13,740	109.05
MT-40	Tube, endotrach., 8	Each	1,620	1,760	108.64
MT-80	Tube, Yankauer	Case	112	123	109.82
MU-40	Underpads	Case	400	462	115.50
			Total		1063.44
			Divided by		10
			Index		⑴06.34

Table 13-3 Total Costs Worksheet for Medical/Surgical Supplies

Stock No.	Base × Quantity	Base Price	Total Dollars	Current Nonbase × Quantity	Nonbase Price	Total Dollars
MB-130	216	$21.50	$ 4,644.00	251	$21.50	$ 5,396.50
MG-65	408	16.41	6,695.28	356	17.44	6,208.64
MH-20	158	44.00	6,952.00	194	75.00	14,550.00
MM-07	1053	6.248	6,579.14	956	6.614	6,322.98
MR-05	98	27.00	2,646.00	98	25.62	2,510.76
MS-47	88	74.33	6,541.04	91	82.44	7,502.04
MT-24	12600	0.33	4,158.00	13740	0.30	4,122.00
MT-40	1620	1.97	3,191.40	1760	2.07	3,520.00
MT-80	112	33.00	3,696.00	123	33.00	4,059.00
MU-40	400	25.00	10,000.00	462	31.25	14,437.50
Totals			$55,102.86			$68,629.42

$$\frac{\$68,629.42}{\$55,102.86} = 124.6 \text{ percent increase in total dollars}$$

Recognizing this problem, Donald Hagen, director of materiel management for the Sisters of St. Mary, St. Louis, Missouri, has developed a set of formulas to provide a more accurate measurement of the total cost problem. This calculation begins by establishing the percentage of total change between the base and nonbase period using the following formula:

$$\frac{\text{Total costs for all items (PNB} \times \text{QNB)}}{\text{Total costs for all items (PB} \times \text{QB)}} \times 100$$

Table 13-3 illustrates this calculation.

The procedure now moves to the price index. In the previous methodology, we established the change by line item. By adding the individual changes and dividing by the number of items that composed the index, we arrived at the average index. With this second method we move toward the effect of individual costs on the total costs. The formula for calculation of the total price index now becomes:

$$\frac{\text{PNB} \times \text{QNB}}{\text{PB} \times \text{QNB}} \times 100 = \text{Total cost price index}$$

Substituting the necessary figures from Tables 13-3 and 13-4, the price index is now determined to be:

$$\frac{\$68,629.42}{\$58,767.98} \times 100 = 1.168 \times 100 = 116.80 \text{ total cost price index}$$

Table 13-4 Total Costs Worksheet for Medical/Surgical Supplies

Stock No.	Nonbase × Quantity	Base Price	Total Dollars	Base Quantity	× Nonbase Price	Total Dollars
MB-130	251	$21.50	$5,396.50	216	$21.50	$4,644.00
MG-65	356	16.41	5,841.96	408	17.44	7,115.52
MH-20	194	44.00	8,536.00	158	75.00	11,850.00
MM-07	956	6.248	5,973.09	1,053	6.614	6,964.54
MR-05	98	27.00	2,646.00	98	25.62	2,510.76
MS-47	91	74.33	6,764.03	88	82.44	7,254.72
MT-24	13,740	0.33	4,534.20	12,600	0.30	3,780.00
MT-40	1,760	1.97	3,467.20	1,620	2.07	3,353.40
MT-80	123	33.00	4,059.00	112	33.00	3,696.00
MU-40	462	25.00	11,550.00	400	31.25	12,500.00
Total			$58,767.98			$63,668.94

Moving to the use index, the new formula now becomes:

$$\frac{(PNB)\ (QNB)}{(PNB)\ (QB)} \times 100 = \text{Use index}$$

Again, substituting the resultant total dollar figures from Tables 13-3 and 13-4, the use index now becomes:

$$\frac{\$68,629.42}{\$63,668.94} \times 100 = 1.078 \times 100 = 107.8$$

Returning to our original logic that the base plus change in price index plus change in use index equals change in total dollars, we can see that

$$100 + 16.8 + 7.8 = 124.6$$
$$124.6 = 124.6$$

At this point, it is important to clarify the calculation methodologies. The first set of calculations was used to measure the average effects of price and usage changes for the sample commodity. The second set of calculations was used to measure the effects of price and usage as they relate to total costs. This is a more exact measurement than the averaging index method.

The development of indexes brings up another problem of which the user should be aware—what to do when an item is added to the index or when an item is replaced. The possibility of this occurrence increases greatly when the ABC method of item selection is used. When a new item is added that does not replace another item, determining the base period price becomes a problem. When calculating statistics of this type, it is an acceptable practice to assume that the base period price for the new item would be equal to the current price divided by the overall price index for the current period. To illustrate this procedure, assume a current price index of 111 percent and a unit cost of $8. The base price for the new item then would be

$$\frac{\$8.00}{1.11} = \$7.207, \text{ or } \$7.21$$

WEIGHTED INDEX

When developing certain commodity indexes, you may want to determine the impact of price changes on a larger group of items. For example, suppose you want to determine the impact of various manufacturers' price increases on the total inventory. To illustrate this point, Table 13-5 shows a listing of specific manufacturers and their respective annual total dollar volume of purchases. Each manufacturer's expenditures represent a certain percentage of total purchases. For example, C. R. Bard's $65,000 represent 13 percent of the total annual dollars of $500,000. To determine the impact that each manufacturer has on the inventory, the percentage of total dollars is multiplied by the latest price index (in this case, the latest price increase). The total of these calculations provides you with a weighted index; in the case of Table 13-5, this is 103.5. This type of index provides an insight as to the contribution each manufacturer has on the total dollars expended. As shown in Table 13-5, the combined effect of individual price increases causes the base expenditure of $500,000 to now be $517,500 or plus 3.5 percent.

Table 13-5 Weighted Index on Total Dollars by Manufacturer

Manufacturer	Total Dollars	% of Total	Latest Price Index	Weighted Impact
C.R. Bard	$ 65,000	13.0	1.046	13.6
Davol	9,000	1.8	1.032	1.9
Ethicon	113,000	22.6	1.082	24.5
Hudson	10,000	2.0	1.040	2.1
Johnson & Johnson	53,000	10.6	1.073	11.4
Kendall	21,000	4.2	1.021	4.3
Monoject	34,000	6.8	1.058	7.2
Pharmaseal	22,000	4.4	1.036	4.6
All Others	173,000	34.6	0.980	33.9
Totals	$500,000	100.0		103.5

($500,000) (1.035) = $517,500

When a weighted index is being used, it is important to review the weight assigned to individual items or commodity groups. Usage of various items will change over the course of time, and the impact of this change will require a redistribution of the weights. This calculation can be made by taking the square root of the current weight multiplied by the base weight. For example, if the current weight for Johnson and Johnson (Table 13-5) were to change to 11.0 percent, it would be recalculated as follows:

$$\sqrt{(11)\,(10.6)} \quad = 10.8 \text{ percent}$$

APPLYING THE DATA

Throughout this chapter, we have reviewed the various types of indexes that can be developed. It is important that generalizations be kept to a minimum and that the data used relate to the answers that are being sought. Too often people misuse data to reflect the results they want to appear. This is especially true if the price index data will be used by administration to evaluate the effectiveness of the purchasing department. Adjusting data to fit the needs of the moment is unethical, and in the long run only tends to create more problems than it resolves.

Developed and maintained properly, indexes are valuable tools. To every extent possible, they should be used to provide a basis for future actions. If prices are rising faster than they have in the past, take the actions deemed necessary to correct, or at least slow down, the price rise. If usage figures do not correlate with other hospital activities, find out why. Properly developed indexes can be the strongest weapon a practitioner can have to prove the need for stronger or improved control over departmental inventories. Develop and use indexes. In the long run, indexes will provide you with information to combat many of the problems that arise on a daily basis.

Chapter 14

Ethics

Since the dawn of civilization, mankind strove to develop principles by which to judge certain acts as right or wrong. As civilization continued to develop, these principles, customs, and practices developed with it and became accepted in matters of trade and business. Eventually, they became written laws. It is from this continued development and understanding of right from wrong that the concept of ethics has evolved to become the cornerstone of business morality.

CONCEPT OF ETHICS

The concept of ethics may be defined as a moral philosophy that teaches duty and the reasons for it. During the last six centuries, ethics has been debated as right on the basis of: (1) the will of God, (2) what reason prescribes, and (3) moral judgments as expressions of human emotion. Regardless of the philosophical treatise on which the concept is based, the ethical implications of purchasing must be addressed by every practitioner.

ETHICAL CONSIDERATIONS OF NAHPMM

It can be said that not to know the principles that are operative in your moral judgments is to be naive. To learn to know them is to achieve sophistication. If hospital purchasing is to reach the highest level of professionalism, the ethical conduct of those engaged in the activity must be defined and clarified for all to understand.

Recognizing that the human equation is present in every aspect of health care purchasing, the National Association of Hospital Purchasing and Materials Management (NAHPMM) has developed a code of ethical behavior for the moral guidance of its members (see Exhibit 14-1). This code of ethics was adapted from a code of conduct developed and adopted by the National Association of Purchasing Agents, which recognized the need for such a code for industrial practitioners.

Personal Considerations

Health care purchasing is currently carried on in a glass fishbowl, with the daily transactions of purchasing practitioners there for all to see. The need for personal conduct that is above reproach has become a necessity. The mere appearance of a good moral character and the claim that one adheres to a code of ethics are not enough. Actions speak louder than words, and it is by daily actions that the individual is judged.

Every employee and vendor representative who visits the purchasing department should be treated fairly and equitably. Hospital personnel should feel confident that no one department or request is given preference. Vendor representatives must share the confidence of hospital personnel. There is no room in today's health care purchasing for personal prejudice. The existence of prejudice can only hinder the effectiveness of the practitioner and the department, and the reputation of the hospital. Once personal prejudice is perceived, even if untrue, it can take years to disprove. It is very difficult to communicate that impartiality truly exists in the purchasing profession, and the practitioner must work very hard at convincing everyone of its existence.

Every practitioner must rely on the concept of what is right and wrong—whether something is legal or illegal is not sufficient. A practitioner should maintain the highest of standards, be obligated only to the hospital, and pursue only those items that are in the best interest of the hospital.

Gratuities and Entertainment

Within the purchasing profession, the subject of gratuities and entertainment has received considerable attention. Many essays have been written regarding these topics, yet there is no definitive ethical standard on which to base a decision of what is acceptable and what is not acceptable. Many hospitals have developed written policies prohibiting ''excessive gratuities and entertainment'' for hospital employees. The principal inconsistency with many of these policies is that the term ''excessive'' is not clearly defined. Hospitals that have tried to define ''excessive'' have used monetary values with upper limits of $5 to $10.

Enforcement by the hospital of such policies is practically impossible. Typically, hospitals that have a written policy apply it equally (at least on paper) to purchasing and other individuals who may influence the purchasing decision. These ''other'' individuals include physicians, nurses, department heads, super-

Exhibit 14-1 Code of Ethics

FOUNDED - 1957

National Association of Hospital Purchasing Materials Management

Headquarters Office: 875 North Michigan Avenue—Suite 3744
Chicago, Illinois 60611—(312) 440-0077

WE SUBSCRIBE TO THE FOLLOWING CODE OF ETHICS

LOYALTY TO OUR HOSPITAL - JUSTICE TO THOSE WITH WHOM WE DEAL
- PRIDE IN OUR PROFESSION -

1. To consider, first, the interests of our hospital in all transactions and to carry out and believe in its established policies.

2. To buy without prejudice, seeking to obtain the maximum ultimate value for each dollar of expenditure so the patient may receive the best care possible at as low a cost as possible.

3. To be receptive to competent counsel from our colleagues and to be guided by such counsel without impairing the dignity and responsibility of his office.

4. To respect our obligations and to require that obligations to us and to our hospitals be respected, consistent with good business practice.

5. To subscribe to and work for honest truth in buying and selling, and to denounce all forms and manifestations of commercial bribery.

6. To decline personal gifts or gratuities which might in any way influence the purchase of materials.

7. To avoid sharp practice.

8. To accord a prompt and courteous reception, so far as conditions will permit, to all who call on a legitimate business mission.

9. To counsel and assist fellow purchasing managers in the performance of their duties, whenever occasion permits.

10. To cooperate with all organizations and individuals engaged in activities designed to enhance the development and standing of purchasing in conjunction with sound Hospital Administration.

visors, and administration. Given the wide range of individuals and opportunities, who would really have time to enforce the policy?

The real question to be answered is, what does it take, in terms of gratuities and entertainment, to influence the purchasing decision-making process? Most often, this question is answered by the vendor, and not by the purchasing practitioner or other individuals. It is important to recognize that overt bribery is not being implied here, but subtle actions by the vendor. This subtle influence is exerted through sponsoring local and national meetings, having hospitality suites at conventions, making donations to the hospital, etc. While the vendor answers the question, it is the purchasing practitioner who is caught in the middle and must deal with the problem. Within the realities of purchasing, a double ethical standard appears to exist. The first standard tells the practitioner not to compromise the purchasing position by accepting gifts and gratuities. The second standard says that it is alright for others involved in the decision-making process to accept such gifts and gratuities because purchasing will make the final decision. How does the professional practitioner deal with the problem? This is best accomplished by recognizing that the problem exists and maintaining a high ethical standard that precludes the acceptance of gifts and gratuities. To assume this ethical position is easier said than done, but as the purchasing practitioner, you are the individual who lives in the fishbowl. Acceptance of gifts or gratuities, regardless of cost, will give a lasting impression to the vendor and hospital personnel that your decision-making processes can be influenced.

Conflict of Interest

A conflict-of-interest situation can be described as existing when:

- The practitioner owns stock in a vendor doing business with the hospital.

- A member of the practitioner's immediate family owns stock in a vendor doing business with the hospital.

- The potential awarding of business can influence (either directly or indirectly) the earning ability of an immediate member of the family.

As an ethical practice, such situations should be a matter of record and publicly acknowledged through a letter to administration. From a practical viewpoint, the practitioner should withdraw from the decision-making process in matters relating to any of the situations described, especially when large amounts of money are involved.

OBLIGATION TO HOSPITAL

The code of ethics of NAHPMM clearly emphasizes the purchasing practitioner's responsibility to the hospital. Loyalty to the hospital requires that the practitioner's conduct be highly ethical. The practitioner is responsible for acting in the best interests of the hospital in expending limited financial resources while obtaining maximum value. This concept has been discussed in one form or another in those chapters dealing with procedures necessary for efficient purchasing and inventory management. Obtaining maximum value as the primary purpose of any purchasing activity is properly expressed as an ethical consideration.

Maintaining the confidentiality of information is also an ethical responsibility of the practitioner. This responsibility extends beyond the information relative to purchasing and includes maintaining confidentiality of matters relating to patients, and to other situations that arise in the normal operation of the hospital.

It is also unethical to disagree publicly with established hospital policy. Such disagreement should be discussed privately with an immediate supervisor or the hospital administration.

OBLIGATION TO VENDORS

The relationships of purchasing practitioners and vendors involve many ethical considerations. It is imperative that the practitioner understand the ethical significance of certain circumstances that are part of this relationship.

Equitable and Fair Treatment

The practitioner's first responsibility is to afford each vendor representative a prompt and courteous reception, and to advise representatives of open reception times and appointment policies. Vendor representatives who call without an appointment usually have few complaints about a reasonable wait. They can feel that their reception is less than courteous when representatives who know the practitioner are admitted before they are. Time once lost can never be made up, and time has a monetary value to both the representative and the practitioner.

Every effort should be made to establish and maintain a reputation for fair dealing with all vendors. The purchasing department is the hospital's primary link to the business community. Vendors visiting for the first time will gain an immediate impression of the hospital from the way they are treated by the purchasing department. Therefore, it becomes incumbent upon the practitioner to establish credibility for the hospital. If a new representative cannot be seen immediately, arrangements should be made for an appointment at a later time. All representatives must be assured of a prompt, courteous reception and a fair opportunity to detail their product line. These elements are essential to achieve the objective of fairness to all.

Protection of Unique Ideas

Because of their particular expertise, vendor representatives are often called upon to assist in resolving problems. During this problem solving, representatives often devise unique solutions and ideas, both of which can become a problem for the practitioner. For example, this author worked closely with a number of forms vendors in seeking alternatives to preprinted charge label systems. Having explained my thoughts on the problem, each vendor was asked to research potential alternatives. One forms vendor happened upon a piggyback label that was being used by one of the national airlines and designed a similar system to accommodate our particular needs. The solution also offered considerable cost savings for the hospital. The dilemma that arises from this type of situation is whether to give the order to the originating vendor or to competitively bid the recommendation.

The resolution to the dilemma was to give the originating vendor the order, because it would be unethical to utilize the expertise of the vendor without paying for the creative help received. Vendor representatives earn their living from selling ideas and should be rewarded for providing their service to the hospital.

The next question relates to how much the hospital should be willing to pay and for how long before competitive bidding is used. The basis for resolving this question will be highly dependent upon the particular situation. In the case of the label example, the vendor was given an exclusive until the hospital was informed that the idea was going to be marketed nationally and that the representative had been rewarded by the company for the idea.

As a general guide, the practitioner should consider awarding the vendor the hospital's business for a fixed period of time, say six months to one year. The practitioner should also seek to establish a fixed price for the product that does not exceed a certain percentage over the next lowest competitor with a similar product (assuming, of course, that one exists). Another alternative is to seek to determine the design costs and then reach a monetary agreement with the vendor for a settlement prior to use of the product or idea. This alternative should be used if it is understood that the item is exclusive to use by the hospital and does not have additional market value. If the item has potential market value to other hospitals, this alternative should not be utilized.

Disclosure to Bidders

With competitive bidding, there are always winners and losers. For the practitioner, the hardest part of the bidding process is to inform the losers. As a matter of courtesy and fairness, the unsuccessful bidders should be notified immediately prior to the award to the successful bidder. There is nothing unethical in telling the unsuccessful bidder frankly and honestly why the bid was lost. And although that bidder should not be informed as to the exact price or price difference between the successful bid and the losers, it is acceptable to give the unsuccessful vendor a percentage range between the two prices. For example, if an unsuccessful bidder's price was 10 percent higher than the low bid, the vendor would be told the range was 8 to 12 percent. This approach does not compromise the low bidder and it provides the unsuccessful bidder with a range to use to make adjustments in future bid situations.

Competitive bids should always be considered confidential, except when open bids are used. It is unethical for a practitioner to disclose quotations to other vendors in an effort to reduce their prices. This type of practice will quickly destroy the confidence of all prospective bidders and could result in receiving higher quotations in the future from all bidders to allow for later reductions during negotiation.

Negotiation is another area where truth and honesty should prevail. Deliberate misrepresentation or providing false impressions regarding the quantities involved or condition of merchandise received is unethical. Every effort should be made to ensure that no misunderstandings arise during the negotiation and award. Such misrepresentation can be construed as fraud, which, if proven, can result in voiding of the contract by a court of law.

PERSONAL PURCHASES FOR EMPLOYEES

From time to time, practitioners may be requested by an employee to make a purchase of a personal nature. These types of requests are of two types. The first category is when the employee wishes to use the purchasing power of the hospital to obtain a lower price than the employee could command as an individual buyer. While every practitioner would like to assist a friend and, perhaps, show his/her abilities, there are ethical considerations to be recognized. Purchases of a personal nature are outside the recognized scope of the purchasing department. Without specific administrative authority, the practitioner violates the ethic of loyalty to the hospital in securing maximum value for the expenditure of limited resources (salaries of the staff). The second consideration is that such purchases are a violation of the hospital's not-for-profit tax status. Personal purchases fall into the resale category, and, therefore, require the payment of sales taxes. Jeopardizing the tax status of the hospital is a consideration not to be taken lightly.

The second category is requests for material necessary to provide medical care for the employee or the employee's family, and these fall into a gray area. Technically, they do not violate the tax status of the hospital and so can be considered legal. On the other hand, the material may be readily available from local commercial sources, although at a slightly higher price. As a general guide, such requests of this type should be limited to items of a special nature that are not usually obtainable elsewhere. The storeroom should not be expected to serve as a convenience store for employees, where they can pick up bandaids or other common items. This category definitely requires administrative consideration, and the establishment of a clearly defined policy.

USING BUYING POWER FOR CHARITABLE CAUSES

The need to solicit funds for building programs and capital equipment is a reality every hospital faces on a daily basis. Many hospital administrators believe that soliciting from vendors who do business with the hospital is both ethical and necessary if the hospital is to raise the necessary capital to sustain such programs. For the practitioner, this situation can become an ethical nightmare.

The nightmare begins with a request from administration for the practitioner to draft a letter to all vendors, requesting a specific donation. In some instances, administration clearly indicates that this letter should contain a give-or-else implication. As an alternative to the extreme of give-or-else, the practitioner can also be requested simply to supply a list of vendor names and addresses to the individual responsible for fund raising. The fund raiser sends the letter requesting the donation. Later, the practitioner is requested to "follow up" with those vendors who have not responded by a specific date.

The nightmare continues when administration requests that the practitioner give as much "consideration" as possible to vendors who have made donations. Once caught up in this situation, the nightmare continues year after year.

The implications of the nightmare extend beyond the ethical and into the financial consequences of such actions. From an ethical and business perspective, the result is business suicide. No matter what or how good a cause it may be, the give-or-else implication is equivalent to blackmail.

The simple act of followup with vendors who fail to respond can be construed as a pressure tactic. The request for special "consideration" for vendors who make donations is clearly a sharp practice involving partiality and favoritism. Both are unethical. Clearly, the practitioner is caught between the proverbial "rock and hard place."

However, the practitioner is not the only one with a problem. The vendor has a similar situation. Some local vendors tend to have an established policy of reserving funds to donate to hospitals that serve their employee population. Other hospitals outside the vendor's immediate locale receive smaller allocations. Some national vendors try to maintain the good will of all their customers and charge such donations to overhead. Regardless of whether the donation is small or large, as the vendor's overhead continues to rise, so does the cost of the vendor's product. And what about vendors who have a company policy against donations? Are they to be "cut out" for not donating?

By now the implications of the nightmare should be clear. The question is how to deal with it and keep your job at the same time. The answers, in some cases, are not easy. As a practical matter, practitioners asked to participate in fund-raising activities involving vendors should decline on the basis of ethics. The human equation, being what it is, will be unduly influenced by knowledge of how much has been donated and by whom. This influence can result in decisions being made that may not be in the best interests of the hospital.

The use of give-or-else, even by other fund raisers, is unethical. It is definitely a lack of justice to intimidate by an overt threat to withdraw business those who earn their livelihood through legitimate competition.

When confronted with the idea of "special" consideration for vendors who donate, the best procedure is to use competitive bidding and award business on the basis of established procedures. This practice may not always be successful (your decision might be overruled by administration), but you have the responsibility to carry out the intent of the prudent buyer provisions and an ethical responsibility to achieve cost containment wherever and whenever possible.

As a final thought, it is important to recognize that raising money, especially millions of dollars, is quite a prospect for any administrator. If a hospital is considering approaching vendors for donations, it should do so recognizing the full implications of such actions. For the practitioner, it may be necessary to clarify these implications to administration and the board of trustees. This awesome act alone requires a high ethical character for the practitioner who faces the prospect.

RESPONSIBILITY TO THE PROFESSION

As a profession, health care purchasing practitioners are small in number when compared with their counterparts in industry. Each of us has a responsibility to exchange ideas and share our knowledge with our colleagues. The ethical code recognizes this by requiring practitioners to accept advice regarding the performance of their duties. This can be accomplished only by each of us contributing in every way possible to the improvement of the profession of health care purchasing.

Index

About the Author

EDWARD D. SANDERSON, C.H.P.M., is currently the Director of Materiel Management at St. Francis Hospital, Blue Island, Illinois. He received a B.A. degree from Aurora College, where he majored in social science with a specialization in economics. He has been a practitioner since 1967, when he entered the United States Air Force. He is a member of the American Society for Hospital Purchasing and Materials Management (ASHPMM) and a Fellow in the National Association of Hospital Purchasing and Materials Management (NAHPMM). He has been a contributing author to *Hospital Purchasing Management* and *Purchasing Administration.* In 1979, Mr. Sanderson was a featured speaker at the ASHPMM seminar held in conjunction with the American Hospital Association convention in Chicago, Illinois.

DATE DUE